A Patient-Expert Walks You Through Everything You Need to Learn and Do®

JILL SKLAR is an award-winning writer who specializes in medical writing. Her articles, on subjects ranging from heart transplantation to digestive diseases, have appeared in the *New York Times, Style* magazine, *Digestive Health & Nutrition Magazine,* and other newspapers and magazines. She is a board member of the Michigan chapter of the Crohn's and Colitis Foundation of America and a patient expert on www.RevolutionHealth.com and is the author of *Eating for Acid Reflux* (with Annabel Cohen) and *The Five Gifts of Illness: A Reconsideration.* She and her family live in Huntington Woods, Michigan.

ALSO BY JILL SKLAR:

Eating for Acid Reflux: A Handbook and Cookbook for Those with Heartburn
  (with Annabel Cohen)
The Five Gifts of Illness: A Reconsideration

THE COMPLETE FIRST YEAR® SERIES

Acclaimed books by "patient-experts" for those newly diagnosed with a chronic or life-changing condition, each with a foreword by a medical doctor

The First Year—Type 2 Diabetes (Second Edition) by Gretchen Becker
The First Year—IBS by Heather Van Vorous
The First Year—Hepatitis C by Cara Bruce and Lisa Montanarelli
The First Year—Fibroids by Johanna Skilling
The First Year—Hepatitis B by William Finley Green
The First Year—Crohn's Disease and Ulcerative Colitis (Second Edition)
  by Jill Sklar
The First Year—Multiple Sclerosis by Margaret Blackstone
The First Year—Hypothyroidism by Maureen Pratt
The First Year—Fibromyalgia by Claudia Craig Marek
The First Year—HIV by Brett Grodeck
The First Year—Lupus by Nancy Hangar
The First Year—Parkinson's Disease by Jackie Hunt Christensen
The First Year—Prostate Cancer by Christopher Lukas
The First Year—Rheumatoid Arthritis by M. E. A. McNeil
The First Year—Scleroderma by Karen Gottesman
The First Year—Age-Related Macular Degeneration by Daniel L. Roberts
The First Year—Cirrhosis by James L. Dickerson

THE FIRST YEAR®

Crohn's Disease
and
Ulcerative Colitis

An Essential Guide for the Newly Diagnosed

Jill Sklar

Foreword by Manuel Sklar, MD

Second Edition,
Completely Revised and Updated

MARLOWE & COMPANY ■ NEW YORK

THE FIRST YEAR®—CROHN'S DISEASE AND ULCERATIVE COLITIS,
Second Edition: An Essential Guide for the Newly Diagnosed

Published by
Marlowe & Company
An Imprint of Avalon Publishing Group, Incorporated
245 West 17th Street • 11th Floor
New York, NY 10011–5300

AVALON
publishing group incorporated

Library of Congress Cataloging-in-Publication Data
is available.

ISBN-13: 978–1–60094–022–4
   ISBN-10: 1–60094–022–6

9 8 7 6 5 4 3

Designed by Pauline Neuwirth, Neuwirth & Associates, Inc.

Printed in the United States of America

Contents

CONTENTS

Foreword

by Manuel Sklar, M.D.

INFLAMMATORY BOWEL disease, IBD for short, refers to two forms of inflammatory conditions involving the gastrointestinal tract: ulcerative colitis and Crohn's disease. These diseases are of unknown cause, uncertain course, and are characterized by symptoms of abdominal pain and diarrhea, sometimes bloody. Ulcerative colitis is a superficial mucosal condition limited to the colon while Crohn's disease is transmural and may involve any part of the gut. Although there is no medical cure, considerable treatment is available to control or modify the disease process. IBD tends to strike men and women in their youth, affecting the quality of their life as well as that of their family.

The medical literature is replete with articles and texts written by gastroenterologists or other professionals directed at physicians, rarely patients. This book is therefore unique—written by a patient with her perspective for fellow patients. The author, my daughter-in-law, has suffered from Crohn's disease for eighteen years, and has experienced multiple hospitalizations and five major surgical procedures. She has devoted many hours to learning about this disorder, developing an expertise that would challenge most gastroenterologists. Such is the background behind this book.

The early chapters deal with understanding the problems and method of making the diagnosis, coping with the emotional impact upon learning one has the disease, and ideas regarding assembling a support group such as family, friends, and professionals, with an emphasis on ways to find the right doctor. Next follows accurate and easily understood descriptions of the nature of the disease and possible complications and a thorough discussion of the role of medications—including 5-ASA drugs, steroids, immunosup-pressives, and Remicade—as well as their indications and side effects.

The subjects of sexuality, intimacy, fertility, and pregnancy are intensively addressed, much based on personal experience. The risks of cancer are explored and the need for surveillance explained. Again utilizing her per-sonal knowledge, the author offers helpful and practical advice on how to lead a reasonable daily life. Topics such as shopping, traveling, exercising, and dining out, to name a few, are covered. Most intriguing are suggestions regarding how to contend with hospitalization including how to prepare, what to bring, and how to deal with visitors, nurses, and house staff.

The role of nutrition is well covered. How nutrition affects the disease, what should be eaten, and what should not, the value of fiber, the ele-mental diet, and total parenteral nutrition (TPN) are discussed. Surgical options including ostomy management are described and the pros and cons of various procedures mentioned. Finally, the problem of IBD in children is addressed. School arrangements, relationships with friends and family, medication issues, and growth problems are considered.

I have only skimmed the surface of the information found in this book. It will be of great value to every IBD patient and physicians will learn from it.

MANUEL SKLAR, MD, FACS, FACG, is Chief Section of Gastroenterology, Sinai-Grace Hospital, Clinical Professor of Medicine, Wayne State University School of Medicine. He lives in Franklin, Michigan.

Preface to the Second Edition

FIVE YEARS ago, I took on the challenge of writing the first edition of this book. Believe me, it was a challenge.

Though I was a writer specializing in medical issues and though I had had Crohn's disease for more than thirteen years, there was so much to learn at the time: different medications and how they worked, side effects and how others managed them, different surgeries and when they were appropriate, lifestyle modifications to make navigating this world easier for those with a greater reliance on bathroom issues. And that doesn't touch on such subjects as insurance issues, legal rights, pediatric cases, fertility concerns, and so much more. But I did it. I wrapped up the manuscript, had it published, and thought I was done.

Then, a new medication hit the shelves, then another. I also went through two more surgeries and learned more from those experiences. New legislation was drafted and had to be explained. Statistics changed. New genetic discoveries were announced. In short, it was time for a new edition of the book, which you are holding in your hands.

Despite the addition of about 20 percent totally new and completely up-to-date content and current statistics, the style of the book remains the same. For those of you who are newly diagnosed, start at page one and work your way through it at the prescribed pace, first day to day, then week to week, then month to month. The book is also for those who have been diagnosed for a while and may be facing a complication for the first time or a worsening of symptoms. And it is for those who have been diagnosed for a while but just want to know more about the disease. In both of these latter instances, locate the information you need and read on from there.

Inside these pages, you will find new information in virtually every chapter, including the following:

○ Two new drugs are being used in the treatment of the disease and five more are likely to be approved in the coming months. Information on these drugs, their side effects, and their methods of administration are discussed. Other promising advances in medical therapies—stem cell transplant and apheresis therapy—alternative therapy—probiotics, prebiotics, and synbiotics—are also noted.

○ New legislation was introduced in Michigan, Ohio, Minnesota, and Texas that will allow restroom access in businesses open to the public, meaning that "employee only" restrooms will now be available for inflammatory bowel disease patients if the measures pass. The legislation is already a law in Illinois.

○ More information about the impact of the diseases and their treatments on bone density has come to light, so more information on increasing bone density can be found here.

○ The latest advances in genetic discoveries and how they apply to you are reported here, as is the newest information on diet and how it affects those of us with IBD.

○ The latest epidemiological statistics are reported in the following pages. Statistics regarding a host of other issues have been updated throughout the book.

I have many hopes for you, the reader. I hope that you learn all you can about your treatment options, both medical and surgical. I hope that you develop a team of professionals that you can trust to care for you. I hope that you learn the necessary lifestyle modifications to make your life as rewarding and fulfilling as you always imagined it would be, despite the disease that has now entered your life. And I hope you continue to be inspired to do more and learn more about these diseases, even after you have retired this book to a shelf in your personal library.

As always, I wish you the best of luck and improved health on this journey.

Introduction

CROHN'S DISEASE. Ulcerative colitis. Inflammatory bowel disease. Ileum. Rectum. Colonoscopy. 6-MP, 6TG, 6MMP, 5-ASA. Remicade. Ulceration. Mucosa. Colon. Cecum. Resection. Ostomy. Flare up. Fissure. Abscess. Bowel obstruction. Proctitis. Jejunum. Prednisone. Duodenum.

Before you were diagnosed with **Crohn's disease (CD)** or **ulcerative colitis (UC)**, collectively known as **inflammatory bowel disease (IBD)**, you probably never said very many of these words. That is not unusual. If you were to walk up to people on the street, they would most likely be able to point out where their heart or brain reside, but they would not have a clue as to where the jejunum is located, much less what it does. Ask them further about any of the other words on the list and they might be more lost. Now, however, those words will most likely have a whole new meaning, one you probably never thought they would have, and one you never wanted.

The words above can be scary just as the diagnosis of an incurable illness can shake the strongest soul. Are you frightened? Or just confused? How about sad? These are normal feelings when you have been diagnosed with a chronic, essentially incurable disease. But with education and support, you can feel more confident and content not only about today, but also about the future.

Of course, requesting help may be hard because most of us like to see ourselves as independent individuals—especially since the average CD and UC patient is diagnosed on the verge or in the early years of adulthood. We are supposed to be young, strong, and healthy, right? In the past, when we were sick, we had to take medication for two weeks and then we were better. We used to think that chronic illness was something that happens to the old and infirm, not to someone who is just starting to plan the rest of his or her life.

But it is happening, and it is happening to you. To make matters worse, these diseases are very complicated, affecting not only various stops in the gastrointestinal tract but also other areas of the body such as the skin, the eyes, and the kidneys. Surgery, tests, and several medications can be difficult to manage, much less to grasp on an intellectual level.

While this may seem very overwhelming, you can't really throw your hands up or crawl under the covers forever. You have to learn to accept the disease and to become an active participant in the treatment of it. You can rely on your doctors, but unless you have enormous financial wealth, they can't be around you 24/7. Your family and friends also can only do so much. You need to become more confident of your ability to manage the illness and all it entails.

That is why it is so important that you learn about the medical and surgical treatments—things that will help to manage your CD or UC. No one expects you to become an expert in a day. I certainly didn't. It took me more than eighteen years to get where I am now.

What happened to me

I still remember the words that came out of my mother's mouth in the early morning hours after a surgeon stumbled across a Crohn's disease diagnosis for me. The orderlies unceremoniously dumped me from the surgical gurney onto my regular hospital bed and left without a word, apparently unaware of the pain they caused me. Trying to catch my breath, I squinted at the hospital clock to see what time it was when my mother entered the room.

I asked her what time it was. Without looking at the clock, she said, "It's early. Your appendix was fine but you have something called Crohn's disease. Go to sleep and we'll talk about it in the morning."

Still woozy from the anesthesia and beginning to feel heavy lidded from the gentle relief of the painkillers, I drifted off, thinking, "Thank goodness my appendix didn't rupture." At the same time, I felt surprised—no, a little shocked—to learn that the symptoms I had earlier that day were not what my trusted surgeon, then so sure of himself, had anticipated.

The day of February 1, 1989, had started with a Jane Fonda workout tape—remember those?—and a big bowl of raisin bran cereal. Three years prior to this day, I had been told by my doctor, an internist, that I had irritable bowel syndrome and needed to eat more bran to stave off attacks of diarrhea I had been having. He also had told me that I needed to not add so much stress to my life since that was a factor in this poorly understood motility disorder. A full-time scholarship student who was used to snagging straight As, I lived with my parents and supported myself with a part-time job. Cutting out stress was like cutting out breathing, but I relented. Three times a week, I squeezed an hour with Jane into my packed schedule to help lose the stress.

After a quick shower, I was off to my classes at Wayne State University in Detroit, a half hour drive from my parent's home. Halfway through my conversational French class, the pains hit, a wrenching pain followed by waves of more pain that took my breath away. Maybe I overdid the abdominal crunches, I thought. During my U.S. history class, the pain became stronger and I felt like I was going to throw up. I made it through the class but I couldn't stand up straight afterward. I decided to skip a journalism class and head home. Something told me this was nothing to mess with.

I made it home, barely. I found that it is hard to drive hunched over in pain. Once home, I vomited several times, something I loathe doing. I occasionally joke that I would make a terrible anorexic because I love food too much, and I would make an even worse bulimic because I hate throwing up. This vomiting—however awful it was to do—was different. In the past when I was sick with a stomach virus, I would throw up and feel better. That day, the cramps would not only return but also intensify. I felt like someone was sticking their hand into my stomach near my right hip and squeezing with all their might. It was awful but I had felt this pain before.

Almost two years before this fateful morning, I had been hospitalized with similar symptoms. I was a high school student at the time and thought I might have food poisoning from the cafeteria food. The surgeon who later operated on me consulted on the case, but by that time the pain had started to subside; nevertheless, I spent the night in the hospital for observation and testing. An ultrasound the next morning revealed a small amount of a watery substance above my right ovary and below my intestines. The conclusion: a ruptured ovarian cyst. The treatment: daily birth control pills to prevent reoccurrence of the cysts.

But here I was, two years later, having the same pains again. Knowing I was pretty consistent about taking my medication, my mom figured that this bout was something different and possibly more serious.

"The pain worsened and you were hunched over. You were vomiting bile. You couldn't stand up straight," she told me later. "And you just looked awful."

So she loaded me into the car and took me to the nearby hospital where I took my place in line in a corridor swamped with elderly individuals who were among a mini-epidemic of flu sufferers, all of us with emesis basins in hand. The doctors pressed my abdomen in various places, asking if it hurt more when they pushed it in or when they released it. They took blood samples and asked me how many times I had thrown up. And I waited and waited, still feeling nauseous and crampy.

The surgeon who had taken care of me during my high school emergency room visit came to see me. He told me that I most likely had appendicitis and would have to have my appendix removed that night. Because I was twenty, I had to make the decision as to whether I wanted to go ahead with the procedure.

I started to cry. At this point—aside from the ovarian cyst incident—I had never had anything more serious than strep throat and a couple of broken bones. I had never cut myself badly enough to have stitches. I also had never really had to take charge of any medical decisions until this moment. Physicals were scheduled by my mom and sick visits were usually chaperoned by her as well. But now I was a certified adult, supposedly able to make these monumental decisions on my own. The biggest things I had done to date were open a checking account and vote in the presidential election—and neither of those things carried the risk of death. But the doctor said I didn't really have another choice. Through a blur of tears, I signed the form and went ahead with the surgery.

I remember waking up in recovery to a diminutive male nurse who reminded me of the late actor Hervé Villechaize. However, I was certain this was no *Fantasy Island*. I remember seeing my mom and I remember the pain medication. Then I felt safe enough to sleep.

The following day, my surgeon entered the room during early morning rounds. I was still a little loopy from the pain medication. He told me that when he opened me up the appendix looked fine, which prompted him to look for the source of the pain. He attempted to free my intestines to check for holes or abnormalities that might cause the pain but had trouble dislodging them from their usual spot. Upon closer examination he said that they were not soft and pink like healthy intestines but rather were hard and had the appearance of "red cracked leather." Even though the diagnosis was the inflammatory bowel disease known as Crohn's disease, he removed my appendix so that we would never confuse the two again. The surgeon put me on an antibiotic called Flagyl and said I could begin eating again as soon as I had a bowel movement.

While the surgeon had initially misdiagnosed me, it was the closest any of my doctors had ever come to diagnosing my illness. My pediatrician had missed it when my ankles swelled for no apparent reason at age five; he originally thought it was poor kidney function, but when it cleared up and never came back, he failed to offer a reason for it. Without doing any testing, a family doctor later blamed my persistent diarrhea on the use of antibiotics for a recurring throat infection.

In my teen years, an internist did blood tests for a swollen ankle and tender knee when X-rays failed to show the reason for the abnormal swelling. He said I tested negative for juvenile rheumatoid arthritis and lupus. When the swelling went away, he also gave up searching for an explanation. That same doctor was unable to offer an explanation for a fever I had about four months before I landed in the emergency room that February afternoon. My temperature had shot up to 105 degrees F and, although no cause was found, I was given a course of antibiotics "just in case." In case of what was never explained.

My family also visited a different doctor, an internist who came highly recommended because he taught at a prominent medical school. This doctor listened to my symptoms of fatigue, abdominal pain, and diarrhea and tested me for diabetes. When the glucose test came up within a normal range, he felt around my belly and asked me what my grade point average was. From this, he declared that I had irritable bowel syndrome, hence the fiber recommendation and the emphasis on stress reduction. This method of diagnosis, however, goes against the recommendations of the American Gastroenterological Association which suggests that several tests be given to rule out other diseases like celiac disease, diverticulosis, diverticulitis, gallbladder disease and—surprise—CD and UC.

Of all the doctors I had seen up to that point, not one ever recommended a series of X-rays using a barium solution for contrast. Only one doctor (the one who tested me for lupus) in passing suggested a colonoscopy but said it would be done without anesthesia in his office—a prospect my mother thankfully decided against. No one referred me to a gastroenterologist.

In fact, after I was diagnosed, the surgeon who found the disease continued to treat me. He offered me no information on my disease but assured me that he knew what to do. I took him at his word and followed his discharge nurse's advice to eat more bran because the Tylenol 3 with codeine I was taking for incision pain would slow my bowels. This advice not only didn't work, it caused my narrowed ileum to become obstructed two weeks later.

When the bran caused my second hospital visit in a month, my current gastroenterologist stepped in to consult on the case. He asked a lot of questions and was ready for mine in turn. He recommended a course of action including an abdominal CT scan that my surgeon summarily dismissed, sending me instead for an upper GI with a small bowel follow-through. I suffered badly from the test, spending the afternoon with yet another bowel obstruction, vomiting barium and writhing in pain. That day, my surgeon was history.

After being released from the hospital, I struggled with taking medication for longer than I had ever taken medication. I hated the way the steroids made me feel, I hated missing not only midterms but also three weeks of school, I hated that I couldn't go for pizza and beer with my classmates when I did return to school, and I hated the life the disease had handed to me, filled with pills and blood tests and doctor visits. I welled up with rage that turned to sadness. I felt intense loneliness, not able to talk about diarrhea, abdominal pain, and medicine with anyone who had any idea what I was going through. A psychotherapist who also had Crohn's disease helped steer me in the right direction, but my life was forever altered.

While my story may seem long, it can be typical of the diagnostic process for inflammatory bowel disease. Because the diseases have a variety of symptoms—from abdominal pain to fevers, from swollen joints to kidney stones, from eye inflammation to tender nodules on the skin—it can be hard to pinpoint a diagnosis.

How to use this book

What is important in all of this is that now you also have a diagnosis and can begin to move forward with your life. Coming to terms with having a chronic illness is the first step in the process that includes becoming educated about the disease, gaining empowerment to make choices in medication and surgical options, and navigating the altered course of your life that this disease can force upon you.

I know that it is hard to absorb all of this at once. When I was diagnosed, I tried to pretend for a while that this disease really wasn't affecting me. I actually stopped taking medication at one point, foolishly believing the symptoms wouldn't return. They did with a vengeance and I realized I really needed to learn more about this thing in my gut. Since that time, I have read just about all of the books on the topic as well as hundreds of medical studies on a variety of IBD-related issues.

Because of my experience, I have taken the information that I have learned and assembled it in a way that is easy to grasp. This book will take you through the first year of diagnosis, first day by day, then week by week, and finally month by month. It will add bits of knowledge and coping skills layer by layer, walking you through helpful tips and strategies for negotiating daily life as well as information about the disease and its treatment. It is designed for you to read a chapter at a time, so you can—no pun intended—digest and absorb the information slowly.

Realize, however, that this disease is not a linear progression of symptom A and symptom B leading to result C. You may have started out with a life-threatening symptom or no symptoms at all. You may need absolutely no surgery in your entire life or you may need multiple surgeries. In any case, it is important to gain as much knowledge as possible about the condition so you are able to notice signs and symptoms and participate more fully in the treatment of the disease.

As you gain this knowledge and, hopefully, some confidence in dealing with your illness, the book will delve deeper into issues that may have been previously touched on. So, for example, the ostomy mentioned earlier will be dealt with more thoroughly in Month 4.

Each chapter contains two sections: Living and Learning. The Living portion will focus on things you can't necessarily learn from a medical book or study. This is subjective information gleaned from my experience and from other individuals who also have a form of IBD. For example, at no time have I ever read anything about surviving the prep for the colonoscopy, supposedly the worst part of the arduous test. And nowhere was there information on how to cope with an accident in public. Those are things health professionals most likely don't know about since they haven't gone through it themselves.

I hope you learn from these portions that there are others who have been where you are now and who have survived. I also hope you learn practical tips for daily living and that these impart a certain confidence in being able to handle your disease. Further, I hope that you learn that this disease is a small part of who you are, and that life plans can be made in spite of it.

The other section of the chapter, Learning, contains more of the medical science and history of the disease. This is objective information, drawn from studies, medical textbooks, and numerous other sources. Surgical options, medications and their effects, genetics, and other topics are covered. This differs from the Living portion in that the Learning section will talk about a test and the Living portion will tell you what you can do to make it easier, for example. In some sections the Learning portion will come first while in others, the Living will precede the Learning.

I have tried to make the Learning section as thorough but as easy to understand as possible without insulting your intelligence. That is why a subject introduced in the first sections may not be dealt with until later weeks or months. If you have trouble understanding certain words, you may want to check out the glossary in the back; all words in boldface can be found there.

What you won't get from this book is a prescription. Let me first say that I am a journalist by education and training. Though I write stories about medical subjects, I am not a doctor, nor do I want to be one. Therefore I will not say whether one course of medication or surgery is better or worse for you. IBD is so vast in its scope and so varied in the way that it manifests itself in patients—not to mention that each patient responds differently to medications and treatments—that it would be impossible to write a book recommending a particular course of action. Additionally, so much more is being learned every day from research and clinical treatment that such a book would be outdated by the time it hit the bookstore shelves.

Instead, I have tried to share with you a base of knowledge about current medication and treatment theories. You can then take this information and apply it to the next article you read on a breakthrough medication or treatment that pops up in the media or makes its way to a journal. As your disease evolves over the rest of your life, I hope you will build on the foundation of information you will receive in the pages that follow.

I am assuming that you know little about this disease. Upon diagnosis with IBD, many people are given one-page pamphlets that offer only the basic information. And if you know nothing about the disease to begin with, you may not be in the best place to ask the doctors the right questions about it. In making this assumption, I realize that the book may move more slowly for those who are already somewhat knowledgeable. If you are in this category, feel free to use these portions of chapters as reference material and move ahead to the next Living section.

Realize also that my experiences and the experiences of others in the book should in no way reflect a plan of treatment for you. Again, I am not prescribing a treatment. Instead, these stories serve two purposes: to help you to understand that you are not alone in this and to serve as examples of actual experiences of the situation mentioned. To make a decision for yourself, I strongly suggest that you gather as much information as possible about the symptoms and the medical treatments or surgical options and then take that information to your team of medical professionals to formulate a plan of action.

I also encourage you to use as many resources as you can. Continued learning is essential if you intend to always be on top of the latest advances. Seek out books and professionals, websites, and medical studies. Talk about the disease in support groups and listen to what others have to say. Educate others whenever a chance arises; you never know what it will mean to them. It may help them in the future when they or someone they care about may experience the signs and symptoms of IBD.

Be positive about the future

Life did not end with your diagnosis. I promise you that it will continue. Since I was diagnosed on that cold February day, I finished college, graduating with honors and a degree in journalism and English literature; I married the man who was my boyfriend at the time of diagnosis; I gave birth to my beautiful son; I adopted three dogs; I bought a house; I have experienced different cultures in several foreign countries; and I have developed a very satisfying career as a writer and as an active volunteer.

Sure, the disease has had a profound impact in my life. But the impact has not been entirely bad. As a result of being ill, I developed a greater level of patience with others. I have had the opportunity to meet fantastically compassionate people, in person and on the Internet, I never would have met without this disease. I have learned more than I think I ever wanted to know about the human digestive system. I am more sensitive to personal pain of those who are ill, no matter what their diagnosis. And I realize now what is really, really important in my life, something that usually doesn't happen until late in life, if at all. For these things, I am extremely grateful.

While I wouldn't wish this on my meanest sister, I welcome you to a wonderful community of people who understand you and support your journey. You are not alone.

THE FIRST YEAR®

Crohn's Disease
and Ulcerative Colitis

It's Not
Your Fault

MAYBE YOU were on the gurney in the recovery room after a **colonoscopy,** still reeling from the medication and desperately trying to keep your eyelids open. Or maybe you had the fortune (or misfortune, depending on how you look at it) of being fully conscious in the doctor's office with a physician who told you what disease you had and promptly stuffed your hands full of literature and prescription sheets before sending you on your way. Perhaps you were home when the phone rang and the nurse practitioner read off the test results. Or, like me, you were told as your body wallowed in postoperative pain.

Whatever way you were told of your diagnosis of CD or UC, the information that followed is least likely to have been totally grasped. Maybe you recall words like "chronic," "incurable," "surgery," or "steroids," but didn't understand anything beyond that. Most likely, you weren't carrying a notebook at the time and even if you were, you might not have heard everything you needed to know.

What you may have been able to grasp is that you were in shock. It is totally normal to feel this way, even if you were expecting to be diagnosed with IBD. Being told that you have something incurable or only curable with the surgical removal of the colon can feel like a slap in the face.

Some people are stunned and profoundly saddened by the announcement of a diagnosis of IBD, even if they were expecting it. Sunni's first symptom came in the form of sores in her mouth. Months later, those were accompanied by blood in the stool, a sign that sent her scurrying to a **gastroenterologist.** Although she was betting that the diagnosis would be either IBD or cancer, she was initially very relieved to hear her doctor say "**proctitis.**" However, the same doctor later explained that what she really had was UC.

"At this point, I was numb," she said. "All of my earlier elation was gone."

For some, the diagnosis was a disappointing conclusion to a litany of baffling symptoms. Jenny had her first symptoms at the age of twenty when her temperature rose to 104 degrees F and was accompanied by strong abdominal pains. A surgeon performed an exploratory laparotomy and, finding an **abscess,** inserted a device to drain it. Although the abscess cleared up, she continued to have problems, causing another doctor to remove a part of her **ileum** in the next year. While the pain disappeared, she doesn't remember hearing the words "Crohn's disease" for almost two decades, during which time she continued to have intermittent diarrhea. Finally, at the age of thirty-eight, a colonoscopy and **small bowel series** were performed on her.

"As a result, I was diagnosed as having Crohn's disease and was informed of the medications to treat the symptoms. I declined the medications," she said. "I did not accept the diagnosis very well."

Others see their diagnosis as a relief because a certain diagnosis has been established and treatment has begun. Lynn is one of those. Year after year, she suffered with abdominal pain that doctors in her small town explained away as having a "hot appendix." Doctors excluded that diagnosis after a colonoscopy revealed changes thought to represent UC. When the medical therapy prescribed to treat that condition didn't work, another series of rigorous tests were prescribed and a final diagnosis of CD was made.

"I was relieved that there was something really wrong with me and that there was a way to treat it," she said.

Still more see the disease as a logical progression for them. Usually, these individuals have another family member or members who were diagnosed with a form of IBD in the past. Amy came from a family steeped in IBD. An uncle, two cousins, and a great-aunt either had CD or UC. She developed symptoms shortly after giving birth, not an uncommon scenario. Then, she sought the advice of a colorectal surgeon who was unaware of her family history. A **sigmoidoscopy** was done and tissue samples were taken, confirming a diagnosis of UC.

"Only then did he ask about my family history, also the sexes of who had Crohn's disease and who had ulcerative colitis," she said. "He said that my symptoms made more sense now that I had ulcerative colitis."

Whatever the case, the diagnosis is usually a shock to some degree or another, and that is perfectly natural. You probably weren't feeling well, but whatever it was you thought you had, you most likely didn't think it was incurable or curable only if a big chunk of a major organ was removed. Add to that the fact that you are facing decades of nonstop medication and most likely an occasional major surgery, and it is impossible not to be shocked.

So, for your first day, we are just going to deal with what you have right now: a diagnosis and a bit of shock. Just let that sink in. And as you are going through all of the accompanying feelings—perhaps a bit of denial and certainly a lot of wonder—just remember this next line: there is nothing you or anyone else did to cause this.

You are not to blame

Now, there might be one or two ill-informed individuals who may say that if your diet was better—without so many burgers, fries, or soda pops, and with much more fiber—you might not have diarrhea. Others will say that an addiction to cigarettes could be the root of the problem. Still more will say that the stress that you put on yourself was going to lead to something bad one day or another.

But the truth of the matter is that no one is really sure exactly what causes these diseases. Diet has been looked into time and time again. While some foods and beverages definitely can stimulate the gastrointestinal tract to cause more daily bowel movements, there has been no consistently prescribed diet to counteract the effects of the diseases, not to mention a preventative one. Cigarette smoking has been found to irritate a case of CD but the opposite is true for those with UC; smokers giving up the habit were found to have exacerbations of their symptoms. In fact, some UC patients use nicotine patches to control some of their symptoms. Stress is something that nearly every human being lives with and yet not every human being has IBD. While it can worsen the symptoms, stress does not cause IBD.

There are, however, theories as to what causes IBD. The first has to do with branches of a tree—your family tree, that is. Genetics plays into a number of things that make you who you are. Perhaps, like me, you have your grandfather's eyes. Or maybe you inherited, like my sister, your olive skin from your mom. Your ability to play music or to learn languages easily may be in your genes as well. It only makes sense that these same genes you inherited may have brought the bad with the good.

Many different kinds of diseases are carried through the ages through the DNA of our ancestors. In some families, the same is true for UC and CD. It is not unusual to find that someone who is newly diagnosed is related to someone who is already a patient. Statistics show that risk factor for developing IBD is ten times greater among individuals who are related to someone who has already been diagnosed with it. That number jumps to thirty times greater if the relative is a sibling or parent.

This finding prompted researchers to examine more closely the possibility of a genetic basis for IBD. In late 2006, researchers discovered that faulty coding on gene interleukin-23 receptor found on chromosome 1p31 predisposed people to CD and UC, while different coding may protect others from ever developing IBD. In past years, scientists have determined that a segment of chromosome 16, called the **NOD2/CARD15** gene, may be related to CD. Other researchers found that people with UC had a 41 percent higher chance of having something called antinuclear antibodies than people in the general population, a marker that appears to be genetic.

Since genes are commonly carried in ethnic or racial bloodlines, certain groups of individuals have historically had a higher risk of developing IBD. Ashkenazi Jews—those who are of Eastern European descent as opposed to the Sephardim who descended from Jews who initially settled in more Mediterranean areas—are four to five times more likely to develop either UC or CD than the general population. Caucasians are more likely than other racial groups to develop the disease, closely followed by African Americans, and less so by Hispanics and Asians.

Because you didn't get to pick your parents or your bloodlines, you are not to blame for having this disease.

Genes aside, scientists theorize that there may be other causes for the disease found in certain environments. For example, researchers have examined various bacteria and viruses as the possible causes of IBD. At the same time, other researchers are focusing on the lack of certain substances within developed countries, areas with the highest density of IBD in the population.

Many scientists also feel that a combination of genetics and environment contribute to the formation of IBD. In this case, they feel that the presence of the gene alone is not enough to the onset of the disease. At the same time, environmental factors alone will not account for the presence of IBD. The combination of the two, they feel, is the reason that some people get this disease and others don't.

Again, even if a pathogen is someday discovered to be the cause of either CD or UC, there is nothing you could have known and possibly nothing you could have done to avoid it.

IN A SENTENCE

It is not your fault, nor is it anyone else's fault.

learning

What is IBD?

INFLAMMATORY BOWEL disease (IBD) is a catchall term that encompasses a variety of conditions that are marked by inflammation and can occur anywhere from the lips to the anus. There are two main diseases that are commonly referred to as IBD: Crohn's disease and ulcerative colitis.

What is Crohn's disease?

Crohn's disease was first written about in the United States by Burrill B. Crohn, Leon Ginzburg, and Gordon Oppenheimer, a team of doctors in New York City who noticed that fourteen patients shared the same characteristics of a disease pattern affecting the last part of the small intestine known as the terminal ileum. Their paper on the topic was published in the *Journal of the American Medical Association* in 1932. Later in the same year, the same doctors reported on fifty-two others who also shared some symptoms, specifically the formation of small lesions called **granulomas** that were found in the small intestine.

While Dr. Crohn was the one for whom the disease was named, he was in no way the first to find it. According to Dr. Joseph B. Kirsner, a leader in IBD research and treatment, a physician performed an autopsy as early as 1612 on a boy who had symptoms like those of CD. Another physician, T. Kennedy Dalziel of Glasgow, Scotland, reported on nine cases of "chronic intestinal enteritis" he had seen as a surgeon in a hospital there in 1913.

What are fairly clear are the characteristic markers of the disease in the gastrointestinal tract. CD can affect any site along the entire gastrointestinal tract—the lips, the oral cavity, the **esophagus,** the **stomach,** the **duodenum,** the **jejunem,** the ileum, the **ileocecal valve,** the **cecum,** the **ascending or right colon,** the **transverse colon,** the **descending or left colon,** the **sigmoid colon,** the **rectum,** and the **anus.**

(While you may be scratching your head about many of these terms, most of which you may have never heard, it might be helpful to acquaint yourself as to their anatomical location by using the drawing on page 46 of the digestive system.)

Because of this, the disease may go by other names, which indicate exactly where the diseased portion of the intestines is located. For example, it is commonly located in the ileum where it is referred to as ileitis or Crohn's ileitis or regional enteritis or terminal ileitis; if it involves the ileum and the colon, it is ileocolitis. When it is in the stomach or first few loops of the intestine, it is known as gastroduodenal Crohn's disease. If it is in the next few loops of intestine, it is called jejunoileitis. If it resides in the colon, it is known as Crohn's colitis. Another term for the disease is granulomatous ileitis or enteritis.

Just as Juliet wondered whether a rose by any other name would smell as sweet, a form of Crohn's disease by any other name usually acts the same way. Sores or lesions appear on the surface of the **mucosa,** the innermost layer or lining of the intestines; the mucosa is assigned the job of absorbing salts, water, and other substances while releasing mucous. The different layers of the bowel wall become inflamed, past the muscular layer of the intestines to a protective coating called the **serosa.** Also inflamed at times is the **mesentery,** the semi-circular fold of the **peritoneum** that holds the blood vessels and lymph glands associated with the intestines and adheres to the intestines as a means of support.

Generally, the symptoms of the disease include abdominal pain that can range from cramps to sharp, localized pains; a change in bowel motility such as diarrhea or constipation; blood in the stool, the color of which depends upon where it is released in the intestines and ranges from bright red to black; vomiting; nausea; lack of appetite; fever; fatigue; painful abscesses and resulting **fistulas;** and weight loss.

The disease can also affect other areas of the body such as the eyes, the kidneys, the liver, the bones, the joints, the gallbladder, and the skin through related conditions. Because of this, occurrences such as strange bumps on the skin, reddened or itchy eyes, **kidney stones, gallstones,** and swollen and painful joints can at times be related to CD.

There are a number of medical treatments that are effective in reducing or controlling inflammation in CD patients, and there are surgical options when the medical efforts fail, when abscesses or fistula occur or scar tissue threatens to block intestinal openings. However, there is presently no cure for CD.

What is ulcerative colitis?

Like CD, UC has a history that predates when it was actually named in a medical journal article. In fact, cases have been documented in medical literature for more than two hundred years. However, with the greater presence of dysentery and other infectious diseases, it made it harder for physicians to definitively distinguish between infectious and non-infectious colitis.

One important invention that debuted in 1913, the electric sigmoidoscope, changed the course of the research on the subject of ulcerative colitis, a term that appears in an English doctor's paper in 1859 regarding an autopsy of a woman who suffered from diarrhea and fever. The sigmoidoscope allowed physicians to literally shine a light upon this little known phenomenon. Greater strides were made in the next few decades in separating the cases of ulcerative colitis from those of infectious origin.

What is understood now about UC is that it strikes the large intestine or colon, unlike Crohn's, which affects the entire GI tract. Found from the cecum to the rectum, UC tends to spread in areas that are close to where it begins, not skipping around as CD does at times. It also appears to affect primarily the mucosa and doesn't burrow through the bowel wall.

Named for the areas that it strikes, UC can go by other names such as ulcerative proctitis (affecting the rectum only) and proctosigmoiditis (the rectum and the sigmoid colon). As the disease reaches further up the descending colon to the **splenic flexure** (located at the corner of the

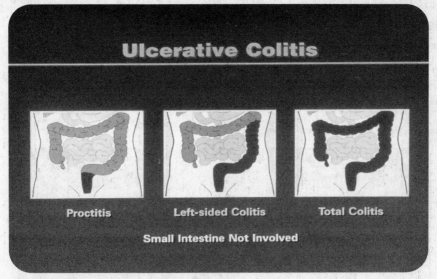

Ulcerative Colitis

Proctitis   Left-sided Colitis   Total Colitis

Small Intestine Not Involved

Unlike CD, UC spreads proximally.

©Crohn's & Colitis Foundation of America (CCFA). Reprinted with permission of CCFA.

transverse colon and the descending colon), the disease gains the name of left-sided colitis. When it takes over the entire colon, it is called panulcerative colitis or total colitis.

The disease manifests itself in the mucosa. Changes at that level lead to the inflammation and ulceration that in turn cause a disturbance in the absorption of salt and water. The malabsorption of the water leads to diarrhea; damage to the mucosa can also lead to excessive amounts of mucous in the fecal matter. The ulcerations cause bleeding, which can lead to **anemia.** Abdominal pain, fever, fatigue, loss of appetite, and weight loss often accompany the disease as well.

Ulcerative colitis also can manifest itself in other areas of the body such as the liver, the eyes, the skin, the joints, and the kidneys, and can account for symptoms such as strange bumps on the skin, reddened or itchy eyes, kidney stones, gallstones, and swollen and painful joints.

There are a number of medical treatments that are effective in reducing or controlling the inflammation process in UC patients and there are surgical options when the medical efforts fail, such as when scar tissue threatens to block intestinal openings. There is a cure for UC that involves surgically removing the colon, rectum, and anus, leaving the patient with a **stoma**, an artificial opening on the surface of the abdomen.

Due to advancements in medicine and medical technology, both diseases now have extremely low mortality rates. One epidemiological study found that overall survival of IBD patients was similar to that of the Caucasion population but CD patients had a small increase in risk of dying from malignant and nonmalignant gastrointestinal causes.

In whom do these diseases occur?

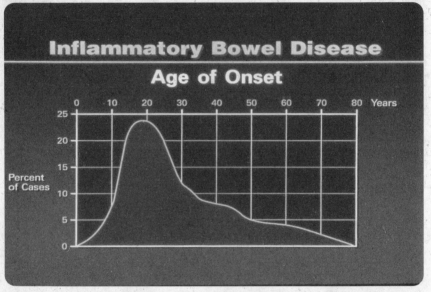

Diagnosis can happen at any age, though is most common between ages 15 and 35.
©*Crohn's & Colitis Foundation of America (CCFA). Reprinted with permission of CCFA.*

At this point, you may feel that you are alone in having this disease, particularly if you have no relatives who have been diagnosed. But you are far from being alone.

One reason why researchers around the globe are frantically searching for a medical cure for these diseases is that IBD occurs globally. People in Australia, Israel, Great Britain, France, Germany, Japan, and a slew of other countries are waking up each day just like you to a regimen of numerous medications.

Epidemiology is the study of the occurrence of certain diseases and other health information in certain populations. Researchers study this information to find disease patterns: information that can show how prevalent a disease is, where more or fewer people have it, whether it is urban or rural in nature, and if certain cultures are more prone to it. Epidemiologists have also studied CD and UC for the past few decades. The information has shifted quite a bit in the past few years, in part due to the increased knowledge about CD and UC that has led to greater ease of diagnosis.

What the epidemiologists have learned is that CD and UC primarily are diseases of the developed world. More people in the Northern Hemisphere than the Southern Hemisphere are reporting cases, and those in the Southern world tend to be in well-developed countries such as Australia. There are also more cases reported in Western civilization than in Eastern civilization.

In the United States, the Crohn's & Colitis Foundation of America did their own in-depth study of occurrence rates and the organization estimates that there are one million individuals with IBD, about 500,000 for each disease; more recent epidemiological studies suggest that the number is closer to 1.4 million in the United States and 2.2 million in Europe for total IBD cases. About 30,000 individuals are diagnosed with the diseases annually. Geographically, higher concentrations of people with the disease tend to be in urban areas as opposed to rural areas. Historically, more cases have been reported in the Northern states as opposed to the Southern states.

Females are as prone to get the disease as males; however, slightly more females have CD over males while slightly more males than females are diagnosed with UC. Disease patterns are not sex-specific; however, women may experience more discomfort and more symptoms during certain points in their menstrual cycles. Some theorize that this is due to hormonal fluctuations that occur during or leading up to ovulation or during menstruation.

As far as age is concerned, CD and UC do not discriminate. The diseases have been diagnosed in toddlers and in senior citizens as well as every age in between. While many believe that CD and UC are diseases of the young, that idea simply is not true. However, physicians say that the incidence is bimodal, meaning there are two general time periods in patients' lives when diagnosis is most likely to happen. The first time is between the ages of fifteen and thirty-five; this is the period of time during which most of the diagnoses occur. About 10 percent of all individuals in the United States with IBD are under the age of eighteen. However, a second though less common time of diagnosis occurs between the fifth and sixth decade of life, making it a disease of the older adult as well.

As reported earlier, people in certain cultures, of certain races, and in certain families are more likely than the general population to develop IBD. Originally thought to be a predominantly Jewish disease, IBD still strikes Jews of Eastern European descent at a rate four to five times greater than the general population. Non-Jewish Caucasians also have a higher incidence rate, though the incidence rate in the African American population has climbed in recent years and nearly matches the incidence rates of Caucasians in many areas of the country. Asians and Hispanics have lower incident rates than both Caucasians and African Americans. About 20 percent of all newly diagnosed individuals are directly related to another IBD patient.

IN A SENTENCE:

> *Inflammatory bowel diseases occur most often in developed areas of the world, in men and women, in the young and the old and in some ethnic and racial groups more than others.*

Grieving:
Are You Sure?

IT'S ALL a mistake, right? Pretty soon, the doctor who shocked you with the diagnosis is going to call you back and tell you there was a defect to the lens piece of the colonoscope and that what he was seeing was not really there. Or perhaps he will say that the lab tests he took to rule out certain bacterial infections were misread and that what you have is a relatively ornery but curable infection that will clear up with two weeks of antibiotic therapy. Of course, you are hanging on to this hope despite the fact that forty-eight hours after your diagnosis you are running to the bathroom more than ten times a day, doubled over with stomach cramps and hoping that the bleeding or the fever won't be so bad this time.

But at least that initial shock is starting to ebb. The good thing about shock is that it eventually wears away. The bad thing about it, however, is that it leaves you with the reality of having to deal with the situation that caused the shock in the first place. And that can be an emotionally trying, grief-filled experience, especially in these days so close to your diagnosis. Let me assure you that this is all to be expected.

The phases of grief

The psychiatrist Elisabeth Kübler-Ross, in her seminal work *On Death and Dying*, found that a terminally ill patient often went through five emotional stages after receiving a terminal diagnosis. For those patients she studied, she wrote that they often experienced denial and isolation followed by anger, bargaining, depression, and finally acceptance of their fate (acceptance will be addressed in Day 3). Since the time Kübler-Ross first reported her findings, many in the field of mental health have ascribed that same emotional pattern to anyone dealing with grief, from a person who has lost a loved one to death to those struggling with a less than deadly disease.

While the findings are common among individuals who are facing a loss through death or disease, they certainly aren't the same for everyone in experience or in duration. For example, I can say, after looking through journals I kept at the time, that bargaining may have lasted one day, tops. Depression, on the other hand, was something I slogged through for months and still haunts me now and then. Others seem to live in denial for decades, never seeming to reach the acceptance phase. Still more gloss over the depression and the denial but have a hard time getting past the bargaining.

But it helps to know a little bit about each of the phases so you know what you can expect and what you might experience. It also helps to know that you are not totally off your rocker for feeling this way. You are not the first to feel this way and you certainly won't be the last.

Denial and isolation

So let's start with a little denial. Denial is defined as refusing to believe a statement despite evidence of its truth. Denying you have a disease when stacks of tests point in no other direction seems a little foolish at first, but it is a self-defense mechanism—something that holds the inevitable at bay until you have the strength to accept it. Family members and close friends may join in the denial process, not because they don't believe what the doctor is saying but because they can't grasp that someone they love is ill.

Denial, like other emotions, does not have a set time limit after which it is supposed to disappear. And, like other emotions, it can manifest itself in various ways. People who are in denial of a CD or UC diagnosis express this through simply verbally denying the disease or by refusing to accept the changes the diseases carry with them such as taking medication. Taking the medication, after all, would mean that the person accepts that they have a disease that needs treatment in the first place.

Six months after the birth of my son, I started having mild symptoms of diarrhea and cramping. I denied to myself that this was happening. Occasionally, blood would appear and I would tell myself that it was due to a **hemorrhoid,** a common occurrence during pregnancy and childbirth. Somehow, I convinced myself that I was fine and didn't need medication anymore. Finally, I could take no more and made an appointment with my doctor. Denying my raging symptoms led to a partial obstruction, which in turn led to my third surgery.

But accepting the diagnosis can be hard. One way to help the denial phase along to its conclusion is to confront the actual diagnosis and question how the doctor or doctors arrived at their decision. It may be beneficial to request copies of all lab work and pathology results from your doctor. Discuss the results and findings with the doctor at length.

Isolation is a little harder to define because the typical definition for it is the separation of oneself from the rest of society. Isolation conjures up the image of a person going off to the hinterlands to die on their own. Loneliness might be a better term. Loneliness is a powerful feeling, not one people embrace easily because it is contrary to the way that most people live. We want to be surrounded by friends and family, especially during times of crisis. Even when togetherness gets to be too much, the times of aloneness are rarely long stretches of days or weeks.

The feeling of loneliness is manifested more internally. For example, you may have a best friend, a spouse, or a parent who accompanies you to your appointments or is there for you in other ways. They may talk to you about the disease or try to gather information for you. But while they are helpful and understanding in every way imaginable, they don't have the disease— you do. This is happening to you and you alone. And that is what makes it so darn lonely.

Jerri was diagnosed with CD when she was ten. She doesn't remember the denial part of grieving. As a child, she seemed more willing to accept having a disease. However, the loneliness of being ill has never quite left her. This feeling seems to arise more when she sees that others don't have to make modifications to their lifestyles when she does. For example, a trip to the lake means nothing to her healthy relatives but she fears having to stop along the way to use a bathroom and won't eat beforehand to avoid this problem. Her loved ones don't entirely grasp her anxiety.

"No one really knows what it is like unless they have Crohn's and this makes me feel as if I am alone," she says. "The biggest for me is the pain. They have no idea what the pain is like and that all by itself makes you feel alone and isolated."

Finding a support group or another individual with IBD can help ease the feelings of loneliness. Simply knowing there is someone else who has been in your shoes—and survived—goes a long way. If there is nothing like that available, speaking with a psychologist who specializes in chronic illness or in grief therapy can also aid.

Anger

Anger usually comes not long after denial has faded a bit. Here, the realities of having a disease that requires medication and possibly surgery have begun to sink in. Swallowing a fistful of pills every day, running to the bathroom frequently or possibly not making it a time or two can set anyone off, either at themselves, at the ones they love, or at the world in general.

A sign that you are in this phase is the oft asked question, "Why me?" or perhaps its variation, "Why not someone else?" Of course, there is no answer to this question. There never has been. Life has no rhyme or reason as to why certain things happen to certain people, no matter how good they have been or how rotten others are. But it is awfully hard to take it in stride when you are angry about something terrible that has befallen you.

When the denial phase ended for Lynn, anger hit full force. Well-meaning people who wanted to help but didn't understand the disease came out of the woodwork, stoking her anger.

"I was angry at the whole world. Why was everyone else allowed to be okay and I wasn't? Why me? What the heck did I do to deserve this? I couldn't be in control of my life anymore. It was controlling me and I didn't like it at all," she says. "I wondered, why in the heck do I have to take all these drugs? What do you mean there is no cure? Am I going to die? Then, there were the people who tried to help but had no clue as to what they were talking about and boy would they really trip my trigger!"

The hardest part about anger is that it is rarely contained within the person experiencing it. Instead, it seeps out on everyone, causing some people to shy away from the angry person lest they become a victim of the misdirected wrath.

A good way to externalize the anger without hurting someone is to practice stress reduction techniques. Gentle exercise such as yoga and tai chi can reduce feelings of anger, as can more vigorous exercise such as kick boxing or running. A regular massage, peaceful meditation, or a long soak in the tub with scented candles burning nearby are other ways people decompress when stressed.

Bargaining

Anger can lead to bargaining, the third stage identified by Kübler-Ross. People with an established religious faith—as well as those whose belief blossoms out of desperation during this period—often turn to a higher power, promising to change or do some good in the world in exchange for a reprieve from CD or UC. Others strike deals with themselves, swearing off some habit and crossing their fingers in the hope that it will make the difference.

What we are really doing when we bargain is simply postponing acceptance until we are more emotionally ready to handle the consequences. Logic tells us that bargaining is futile, yet we do it because we are not yet ready to move forward. For some, there may be a belief that a miracle is waiting for them: if they just ask and offer something in return, it will be bestowed upon them.

Depression

Depression often accompanies just about any disease or sudden change in life. Having to take medication, facing hospital or medical bills, adapting to changes in diet or lifestyle, and dealing with difficult physical symptoms such as nausea, anemia, and diarrhea are all stressful changes people newly diagnosed with CD or UC often face. Depression is a natural reaction to the stress.

Depression may also come from realizing that the chronic symptoms may last a lifetime, separated by remissions that don't last nearly as long as you would like. Unrealistic expectations of what life will be like from now on may be clouded by the difficult symptoms that the patient is facing at the time of diagnosis, leading them to think this new incurable disease will always affect them as it does.

Michelle was initially relieved when a doctor told her that she didn't have CD but that he would like to keep tabs on her situation. When the diarrhea and blood returned, she went back to him. Further testing revealed that CD was, in fact, the culprit. Since that time, depression and anxiety continue to crop up constantly, enough for her to be on prescription medication to combat it.

"When I didn't even think, I was thinking about it. I still do that. My husband and family try to be supportive but I still have days where I feel I'm in this alone. They can't possibly understand," she says. "I have anxiety about my future. Will I be healthy enough to have a good life? Will my children have to witness a sick mother and what effect will that have on them? Will I get fired from my job if I get sick and can't make it to work? There is so much to worry about some days. It's all I can do to stay out of the depression rut."

Some individuals facing depression after diagnosis find solace in attending support groups. Michelle, like others, finds it at an online message board for people with IBD. Others seek private counseling while still more find help with antidepressants or anti-anxiety drugs prescribed by their doctors.

The grieving process is an arduous ordeal for anyone to face. As draining as it seems to be, some people find there are benefits for having gone through it. The important thing to remember is that you don't have to go through this alone. In Day Four, we will discuss finding support.

IN A SENTENCE:

Grief is a process.

learning

What the Tests Tell Us

EVERYONE IS born with a digestive system. In the vast majority of people, it is normal then and for the rest of their lives. For these fortunate souls, their digestive process is the same, day in and day out, meal after meal. You probably counted yourself among them until a couple of days ago.

The normal digestive process

It starts with a food entering their mouth where it is initially broken down by the teeth in the chewing process, known as mastication. Saliva released from the salivary glands along with a squeeze from the muscles we know as the tongue help to push the food into the next step, swallowing. Here, the body uses gravity and a few wavelike muscular squeezes as the food travels literally down the esophagus, a tube surrounded by muscular layers that is located from the top of your throat to your lower chest. You can feel this motion if you place your hand on the front of your throat when you swallow.

At the bottom of the esophagus, the food squeezes through a small passageway known as the lower esophageal sphincter

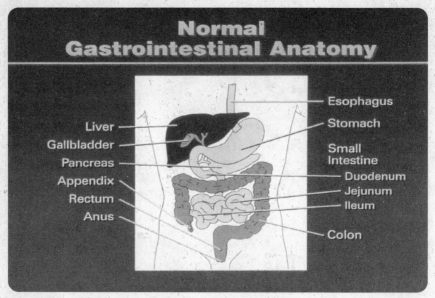

The gastrointestinal tract facilitates an intricate digestive process.
©Crohn's & Colitis Foundation of America (CCFA). Reprinted with permission of CCFA

and into the stomach. There, digestive juices including acid, bile, and enzymes from the liver break the food down to a liquid substance that passes through a muscular structure known as the pyloric sphincter and into the small intestine.

The small intestine is about 20 feet long and looks soft and purplish pink; it is wet and slippery to the touch and rebounds when pressed. It coils around in an intricate heap that is located in the center of the abdomen. These intestines are supported by the mesentery, a semicircular fold of blood vessels and lymph glands, and are surrounded by a sheet of transparent lining called the peritoneum.

When the food passes into the small intestines, it lands in a segment called the duodenum where it is greeted with digestive enzymes from the gallbladder and the pancreas. These enzymes help to break the food down even further so it can be absorbed more readily by the lower loops of the intestine; in particular, **bile salts** and bile acids are released here by the **gallbladder.** The food continues to travel through the small intestines by a squeezing motion, peristalsis, made by a muscular layer of the intestines.

As it passes into the next segment, the jejunum, some of the food that is relatively easy to break down begins to be absorbed through tiny projections in the mucosa called **villi;** these are leaf-shaped in the duodenum and become more finger-shaped the closer they get to the ileum, the last segment of the small intestine. Nutrients like carbohydrates are absorbed higher in the intestines while some elements that are more difficult to break down such as fats, calcium, and vitamin B_{12} aren't absorbed until the ileum. The ileum also reabsorbs bile salts that make their way back to the liver and the gallbladder to help to digest future meals.

The ileum narrows a bit when it joins up with the first part of the colon called the cecum. The spot where the two intersect is known as the ileocecal valve, an opening that helps to pace digestion a bit by slowing the contents of the ileum from pouring into the colon. This area can be felt by placing the right hand about three to four finger widths from the hip bone and pressing slightly.

Finally, the remains of the food—now more liquid than solid—at this point make it to the cecum, the first part of the 6-foot long large intestine or colon. This rounded structure is the home of the appendix, a small, wormlike structure often removed when it is inflamed or infected. The waste travels up through the ascending colon as the colon starts to do its most important task, removing salt and water through the lining of the colon. The waste then makes a right, in an area just below the liver called the **hepatic flexure.** It continues along the transverse colon, located horizontally below the ribs, until it makes another right in an area just below the spleen called the splenic flexure. The waste makes the final descent through the descending colon, a structure felt between the bottom of the left rib cage and the left hip. At about the hip, the colon takes a couple jogs in an area known as the sigmoid colon, a curvy loop of the colon that ends at the rectum. The rectum is a short structure, just inches long, which contains strong muscles that help to hold the waste and then dispatch it through the anal canal and anal sphincter at the appropriate time.

What is normal to one person is obviously not necessarily the same to others. For the most part, a normal bowel movement will not cause tremendous pain, just an easy tension that passes as the fecal matter is discharged. There may be some visible mucous but no blood. For the most part, it will be a shade of brown, not pale yellow or white, and may at times have noticeable particles of undigested matter, such as the corn eaten the night before or seeds from a bowl of raspberries. The fecal matter will be relatively round in diameter, firm but not hard. It will sink to the bottom of the toilet, not rise to the top. Some air may be passed at the time of the movement.

What isn't normal?

This question may have prompted an individual to seek medical attention in the first place. There may be blood on the toilet paper or in the toilet bowl. The amount varies from person to person. A few drops can send some people straight to the doctor while others won't notice until the bowl fills with blood. Or maybe there is excessive abdominal pain and cramping, not only during a bowel movement but also accompanying digestion. A change in the pattern or consistency of bowel movements such as having diarrhea or constipation is also not the norm and should be checked out. Nausea and vomiting are also a cause for concern, especially if these conditions persist.

How do doctors know it is IBD and not some other GI disease?

How a doctor treats a patient when they first complain of these symptoms depends on what the symptoms are and how serious they appear to be. A doctor may not be as concerned about a person who has intermittent diarrhea as they are about a person with a low hemoglobin count, a tender point on their abdomen, and a high fever. The amount and types of tests ordered depends on severity and variety of the patient's symptoms.

And remember, not all of the symptoms will point to just one disease. Diarrhea, abdominal pain, and fever are symptoms shared by a host of diseases, including celiac sprue, colon cancer, gallbladder disease, diverticulitis, **ischemic colitis, C. difficile,** other bacterial infections and irritable bowel syndrome. To make a definitive diagnosis, the diseases must be eliminated from the list of possibilities through testing.

A starting point for every doctor examining a patient for the first time is to take a physical history of the patient. This includes weighing the patient, measuring height, and taking blood pressure and pulse rate. The patient is also asked a series of questions about their health in the past and in the present, including any problems that may run in the family.

Questions about when the symptoms started may help the doctor to determine if the problem is bacterial in nature or not. For example, if your symptoms started not long after you attended a family picnic where your Aunt Alice served potato salad that had steamed to room temperature in a hot car before you ate it, you may have a bacterial infection that is wreaking havoc on your gut.

During a physical exam, the doctor will also palpitate the abdominal region. A physician does this to feel for masses in the abdomen and literally feel areas that might cause pain. An abscess, for instance, may cause sharp pain when it is pressed even lightly. Knowing where this physical pain is located will indicate to the doctor what tests might be needed.

Unfortunately for IBD patients, there is no one single blood test or breath test or stool culture that tells the doctor with 100 percent certainty that a person has IBD; there are serological markers but other tests must be done for confirmation. For now, a doctor must use endoscopic techniques, barium X-rays, blood tests, stool cultures, magnetic resonance imaging (MRI) and **CT scans** or **ultrasound** in combination or alone to rule out other diseases and confirm an IBD diagnosis.

Here are brief descriptions of the tests mentioned above. For more on the topic, see Month 5.

Endoscopic procedures involve the use of a relatively small, snakelike tool that is outfitted with a lens piece, light, and fiber-optic camera that allows the doctor to see inside the GI tract. Where the doctor is looking gives the name of the test. For example, during a colonoscopy a physician will view the colon but in a gastroscopy the doctor will look at the stomach. The device is inserted into either the mouth or the anus and allows the doctor to see inflammatory changes on the surface of the intestines. UC can look like bright red, raw skin, while CD usually has a cobblestone appearance due to its characteristic granulomas. Scar tissue for both appears as white lines or patches. The endoscopic tools also allow the doctor to take a small sample of the bowel wall to be examined later for cellular changes that are indicative of CD or UC.

A relatively new endoscopic method used in diagnosing CD is the endoscopic camera pill. This device, which was approved for use by the FDA in 2001, involves the patient swallowing an endoscopic camera that is in the shape of a pill, approximately the size of a multivitamin. Inside the pill is a tiny camera, batteries, a light, and a transmitter; the patient also dons a receiver, which is stowed in a belt worn around the waist for the duration of the day. As the pill is propelled through the upper digestive tract by normal digestive muscular movements, it takes thousands of photographs and transmits the images to the receiver. At the end of the day, the information is downloaded into a computer for the doctor to read the images, some of which can show tell-tale signs of CD.

A barium X-ray series may also be ordered. During this X-ray, a radiologist will either insert barium into the colon through a tube that travels through the anus into the rectum or have a patient swallow a few glasses of barium and then take a series of X-rays as the barium highlights certain normal and abnormal occurrences in the GI tract. At times, air is pumped into the GI tract during these tests to provide a second contrast. The radiologist will then consult on the findings with the doctor ordering the test. Various images can appear that would point to a diagnosis of either CD or UC.

An ultrasound primarily is used to visualize the gallbladder and liver but is at times used when a patient is too ill to prepare for or too weak to withstand an endoscopic procedure or a barium X-ray series. An ultrasound technician will apply a gel to the abdomen and use a wandlike object on the skin. The wand uses sound patterns that bounce off the internal structures, which in turn provide a picture of the structures that are projected onto a monitor. While disease activity can't be seen on an ultrasound, a thickened bowel wall can be detected and other potential causes of abdominal pain can be eliminated. Usually, further testing is done at a date when the patient can withstand it.

A CT scan is a tool that is used to detect the presence of abscesses in the GI tract. The device is a large hollow tube that has a table that slides in the middle on which the patient reclines. A contrast solution can be dripped in intravenously or can be swallowed to allow the internal structures to be highlighted. Images produced by the machine are cross sections that allow the doctor to see if there are abscesses, which appear bubblelike.

Another quick series of tests a doctor can order involves taking a small amount of blood or stool. The stool is collected in a small cup and then examined for the presence of parasites or their ova, for the presence of blood or for the presence of certain bacteria or viral components. A complete blood count tells the doctor if the white cell count is elevated or if the hemoglobin is low, two things that typically happen in an IBD patient. An erythrocyte sedimentation rate can indicate inflammation in the body. A metabolic panel allows the doctor to see how the liver is functioning.

Further, more specialized blood tests can also be done to detect the presence of certain markers in the blood that are common for people with IBD and to further detect specific components for UC or for CD. These tests are not 100 percent accurate for the presence of IBD and should be used in conjunction with other diagnostic methods.

What is ruled out and how is it ruled out?

Now, the doctor has all of the test results. How do they differentiate between those other GI conditions mentioned before? Let's go through them, one by one.

Celiac sprue is a disease that is caused by an immune reaction to gluten, a wheat by-product. Since wheat is in not just bread and pasta but everything from ice cream to ketchup, celiac sufferers might have diarrhea and abdominal pain anytime they eat. This condition is diagnosed by a definitive blood test that detects antibiodies to gluten; a **biopsy** of the ileum showing flattened villi can be helpful as well.

Diverticulitis is a condition marked by the formation of pouches through the outer wall of the intestines. The pouches themselves are not dangerous unless they become infected, inflamed, or perforated. More common as humans age, the pouches can be seen during a colonoscopy but also appear on a barium X ray.

Colorectal cancer can be present in a patient with no symptoms or it can cause a change in bowel habits, the presence of blood in stools, and the onset of abdominal pain and cramping. Fecal occult blood tests can confirm the presence of blood but further endoscopic or radiologic tests such as the lower GI, colonoscopy, or sigmoidoscopy are more beneficial to the physician making the diagnosis. Colon cancer can look like a bump on the mucosa, a discolored spot, or a **polyp.** The disease is confirmed with a biopsy.

Gallbladder disease can start out with symptoms that are similar to pain that comes with a bowel obstruction—deep wavelike pain, nausea, and vomiting. Stones formed from cholesterol in the gallbladder block the path of bile to the duodenum, causing a squeezing motion to follow as the gallbladder struggles to free the blockage. Usually, the disease happens in people who are over the age of forty, overweight, pregnant, or from certain ethnic backgrounds, such as the Pima Native American tribe. It is confirmed with tests such as an ultrasound, HIDA scan, or isotope study.

Ischemic colitis is caused by a disruption of the flow of blood to the colon. It produces many of the same symptoms as IBD such as diarrhea, blood in the stool, fever, nausea, and vomiting. More common in people over fifty, this form of colitis can be visible during a colonoscopy and confirmed through a biopsy. An arteriogram—a study of the arteries using a contrast solution—can show lesions that would indicate a blockage of blood flow.

Clostridium difficile, or C. *difficile*, is a bacterium that is found in the fecal matter of humans and animals. When antibiotics are used, bacteria levels in the colon change, which can lead to diarrhea. Other bacteria such as campylobacter or E. *coli* also cause changes in bowel patterns, bleeding, abdominal pain, and fever. A stool test can determine if this is the cause of the diarrhea.

Irritable bowel syndrome is a motility disorder that causes changes in bowel function such as diarrhea, constipation, or both. Stress and diet can affect the individual with IBS. Because there are no physiological manifestations of the disease such as inflammation and scarring, IBS is not seen using endoscopy or barium X-rays. Usually, the diagnosis is rendered when no other disease process can be found.

Talk with your doctor about the findings that he or she has made. Ask about how these findings point to a diagnosis of CD or UC. The more you know about the disease in your body, the better equipped you will be to be a partner in the treatment of it.

IN A SENTENCE:

> An IBD diagnosis is made based on the results of tests that also rule out other conditions.

Acceptance
and Hope

IT IS the third day since your diagnosis and we are talking about acceptance and hope. You, however, may still be in shock or in denial mode. That's okay. It is going to take a while to get to acceptance. But for today, let's learn a little bit about what lies ahead of you.

Acceptance, the destination of grief's journey

At the risk of sounding too New Agey, I believe that grief is a journey filled with emotional phases. The destination of the journey is acceptance and stops along the way are the stages we discussed in Day 2: denial and loneliness, bargaining, anger, and depression. And the partner you take with you in all of this craziness—the thing that buoys you even as you feel your worst—is hope.

As a certain domestic goddess might say, acceptance is a good thing. Acceptance is defined as the act of taking what is given or offered. It usually happens after you have dealt with denial, let go of most of the anger, stopped bargaining, and begun to grapple with depression. It does not often come without a struggle that lasts a few months to a few decades.

Acceptance is the part of the grieving process when the darkness of the disease gives way to the light that you feel when you are in control of your destiny, at least to some degree. There is a certain peace that comes with acceptance as the difficult emotional struggle takes its toll.

You may feel like you are there when you are able to explain why you have to rush to the bathroom or why you order certain foods while dining out, saying "I have IBD." It takes courage to accept your destiny with IBD, moreso to tell others. While people may openly discuss their latest bypass surgery or be lauded as a heroine for surviving breast cancer, IBD is one of those diseases that people infrequently talk about because the symptoms (rectal bleeding, diarrhea, vomiting, etc.) make for uncomfortable conversation at best. We were taught as kids that diarrhea is embarrassing (remember those rhyming songs about it?), that "anus" was a funny word, and that discussing bowel habits was rude. Overcoming these social stigmas and being able to discuss them openly with others is a leap forward.

You may feel that you are close to acceptance when you finally begin to crack books on the subject of inflammatory bowel diseases, seeking out information instead of having some family member foist it upon you in an effort to do something, anything, after you are diagnosed. Educating yourself about the disease is a step toward acceptance, and education allows you to be a knowledgeable partner in the treatment of the disease. Having knowledge about the disease allows for you to be in a greater position of control.

You may feel that you are there when you begin to ritually and willingly take your medication. Another step here is to schedule and keep regular appointments with your doctor so he or she can measure your progress and deal with any emergent issues such as fevers or the onset of new symptoms. Taking your medication and seeing your doctor regularly indicate cooperation in caring for yourself, something you may not do as freely if you were still in denial of having the disease.

Accepting the disease does not mean that you will not occasionally feel some of the feelings you have passed through to get to this point. Denial can return if you have had no symptoms for a really long time, just as depression can rear its ugly head when symptoms return during a flare-up of the disease. Instead, it means that you are ready to move on with your life, disease and all, even if you sometimes return to some of the stops on grief's journey.

Hope, a constant companion

Hope is different from acceptance. It is desire married with expectation. Hope can be rabidly intense, something to cling to when the worst is all about us, but it can also be quiet and ever present, a soothing companion during these darkened periods in life. Hope allows us to soar when in reality we are closer to crashing and it keeps us going when we would rather quit. But one of the most wonderful aspects of hope is that it never seems to leave us and even when it may, it is never too far away to retrieve.

For those of us with IBD, hope comes in many forms. Hope is that flutter you feel when you are holding your breath and taking that X-ray, the thought present in the back of your mind that the radiologist won't find anything significant this time. Hope is what causes you to cross your fingers as you wean from **prednisone** and wish that you never take it again. Hope is the flicker in your eye when you read the latest development of a drug that passes into the next phase of FDA trials or some discovery a scientist has made. Hope is the participation in the search for a cure.

Telling others about your condition

Whether you are armed with acceptance and hope at this point or not, you will have to get back to reality, and that may mean having to tell people something. What that something is is really up to you. How comfortable you are right now will determine not only whom you tell but also what you tell them.

I never hesitate to tell people about my CD. I don't introduce myself and then corner a new friend with gory details of CD, but I don't hide it either. Usually, it comes up because I have had a fever or some other symptom that has made me a tad less mobile and I have to explain that what I have is not contagious. My friends all know, mostly for gastronomic rather than gastrointestinal reasons; they realize that if we meet for lunch or dinner, we have to pick a location that serves fish or vegetables that aren't fried and has more than one bathroom stall. During times when I am particularly under the weather, I often find myself telling more people, in part because some ask what terrific diet I am on to lose so much weight, or they invite my husband and me to join them on an outing. I have told the other mothers who have children on my son's soccer team so that they can watch Jonah in case the need for a quick potty trip arises. On the same note, my son understands that his mom has a greater need for the bathroom and often joins me on the hunt for one when we are out in public; he hovers over me when I don't feel well and has said that someday he wants to be a "tummy doctor" to help me. My family has known from the beginning and they are pretty much sick of hearing about it by now.

As a freelance writer, I tell the people with whom I am under contract that I have CD only when the need arises. For example, I told one editor that I couldn't do a story because I was recuperating from having a **resection** earlier that week. The disclosure led to a short discussion, during which he told me that he had the same bowel surgery the year before. He later called to see how I was healing and to offer me another story with a more manageable deadline.

But not everyone is so open, especially when they might still be struggling to accept the disease themselves. Talking about the disease brings up that social taboo of discussing bathroom habits in public, a difficult position for some to overcome. People also often don't tell others about it because they expect that the person they tell will show pity for them.

The head of the household or the major wage earner in the family may have a more difficult time divulging their diagnosis to the rest of the family. Men in particular may struggle with telling their loved ones of their diagnosis because of society's view that men are the stronger sex; in this vein, any admission of illness is equated with weakness.

Caretakers are another group of people who have a hard time telling loved ones that they are ill. When you are always the one who takes care of others' needs, it is hard to change roles and be the one who is sick. If you are a parent of smaller children, it may be especially trying to tell your family members of your illness. Illness can be frightening to children; when illness strikes their parents, children can become anxious and knowing this can make it harder for the parent to tell the child.

How to tell people about the illness depends on how much information is needed and that will be something you determine on a case by case basis.

Some people may not need all of the details. For example, you need a baby-sitter to watch your kids while you run to the doctor for an appointment. The sitter really only needs to know when you are coming back and a number where you can be reached. Therefore, giving that person a blow by blow account of the disease, your personal medical history, and the quantity and quality of your bowel movements may be too much information or scare them away. But letting that same sitter in on the details (perhaps leaving out the quantity and quality bit) when you are planning a hospitalization may not be a bad idea in case the children should have some questions.

When you do tell people, be prepared for the questions they might have about the condition, the medication, and the effect of the disease on you. If you have the answers for their questions, great! But if you don't, tell them that you will ask your doctor during the next visit or suggest to them that they help you find the answer to their questions in books or on the Internet. Beware, however, if they start to act like your personal bodyguard, checking every morsel that passes between your lips or reminding you to take your medication every hour. Realize they do this out of love or caring and then tell them to take a hike.

IN A SENTENCE:

> *Acceptance is the goal in the grief process while hope is the constant partner.*

learning

The Workplace, the Law, and IBD

WHILE TELLING family and friends may not be such a hurdle to most people, cluing in your boss or coworkers is entirely another matter. Unless you work for your relatives, those you love can't jeopardize your job by knowing that you are ill, but your boss or your co-workers can.

Bosses are funny about illness. Some of them can be the best possible people in the world to tell. They watch out for you, make allowances for you when you don't feel so hot, and cut you some slack when you need it. These bosses are the best people to have on your side during hard times.

Michelle has a boss like this, a warm, caring, and support-ive woman who has stood by her from the day she was diagnosed.

"I had no problems talking with my boss because she is just very supportive of everyone in the office and I felt she had to know in case I needed to be off work at some time," she said.

Other bosses believe that a sick employee is a bad employee, one who will rack up more sick time while using and abusing the Family and Medical Leave Act allowances. They think that all of your expensive medication (at least one that could cost about

$3,000 a dose every six weeks) and hospitalizations force up the price of medical insurance for the company. Or they may think that the disease will preoccupy you, causing you to perform at a lesser capacity.

Like bosses, coworkers can save you or crucify you. On the positive end, they can shield you from the boss, carrying you on days when you need a slower pace. But coworkers may resent you for the same reason, claiming they shoulder the slack even if you more than make up for any temporary shortfall in productivity. These individuals are more likely to conspire against you, registering complaints that are exaggerated and mean-spirited with the boss.

Ideally, we would all have the dream boss and the dream coworkers. But sometimes, we are left with less than the ideal. Under these circumstances, it is perfectly natural to not want to tell your bosses and coworkers about your illness. Unless you are suffering obvious, sustained, intense symptoms, you may decide to adopt a "don't ask, don't tell" policy. Either way, telling these individuals is an extremely personal matter, one only you can decide and even then on a case by case basis.

The good news is that right now you and your job are likely covered by laws designed to protect people with ongoing illnesses and disabilities from workplace discrimination. In America, several states have adopted laws that protect worker's rights, safety, and compensation. A handful of federal laws also provide benefits.

There are two such federal laws that provide at least some measure of direct protection and provisions for people with chronic illnesses such as IBD: The Americans with Disabilities Act of 1990 and the Family and Medical Leave Act of 1993.

The ADA

The Americans with Disabilities Act (ADA) has been amended since it went into effect and has morphed through numerous interpretations through the courts in the past decade. The relevant parts of the act for you lie in the definition of a person with a disability and the reasonable accommodations that an employer must take during your employment.

The ADA defines a person with a disability as someone who has a physical or mental impairment that substantially limits one or more major life activities, has a record of this impairment, or is regarded as having this impairment. For the purposes of this book, we will discuss the physical impairment, defined as "Any physiological disorder or condition, cosmetic disfigurement, or anatomical loss affecting one or more of the following body systems: neurological, musculoskeletal, special sense organs, respiratory (including speech organs), cardiovascular, reproductive, digestive, genitourinary, hemic and lymphatic, skin, and endocrine." All individual ailments are not listed as it would be impossible to do so. Clearly, IBD would fit into the protected disorders as it is an ongoing, digestive disorder.

The act also states that the impairment is a disability as long as it substantially limits a major life activity as compared with the ability of an average person. There are three factors that are considered in determining whether the impairment substantially limits the life activity: the nature and severity of the impairment, the duration the impairment is expected to last, and the expected impact. The reason for this wording is that diseases affect people differently, having greater or lesser impact over more or less time depending on the individual. People with lesser impact from their impairment or a temporary impairment may not be covered by the act.

The act protects people who have a record of a disability from discrimination. This means that if you have an active disease or disease that is in remission, your employer can't discriminate against you. Also, if you are regarded as having an impairment, protection is offered by the act. Here, an employer can't discriminate if he or she perceives that the disability is substantially impairing, even if it isn't; if an individual has an impairment that is limiting only because others believe it will be; and if an individual has no impairment but is regarded as having one. One example of this last part is if an employer transfers you to a lesser job, although your IBD is in remission, because the employer fears you will need to be in the bathroom more often. The employer has perceived a greater disability than exists and therefore may be liable for damages under the act.

The protection of the ADA begins the moment an employer becomes aware of the condition. Therefore, it is not a good idea for an employer during a job interview to ask you about your abilities or disabilities except as they pertain to the job. If they do ask and they don't hire you, they may be liable under the act to compensate you not only for lost wages and future wage earning losses called compensatory damages, but also for damages related to emotional pain and suffering.

Another key to the act is that the person who is deemed disabled under the act must be able to perform the job. According to the act, an individual "must satisfy the requisite work, experience, education and other job-related requirements of the employment position such individual holds or desires, and who, with or without reasonable accommodation can perform the essential functions of such position." In other words, if I am looking for a job and have a bachelor's degree and two years experience when the job requires a master's degree and five years experience, I can't invoke the ADA protection just because I fit the requirements for a disability.

"Reasonable accommodation" is a term that also pops up in this piece of law. If there is an individual who is otherwise qualified for a job but can't perform one of the job responsibilities due to the impairment, an employer must make modifications or adjustments for these individuals to do these tasks. For people with IBD, this may mean something as seemingly minor as allowing extra bathroom breaks or having easier access to a bathroom.

If you feel you have been discriminated against in violation of the ADA, there are a few steps you can take to establish a case and protect your rights. First, you should consult your employee manual, if there is one. This should establish a chain of command and a process for giving redress for complaints. Next, in writing, tell your employer about the problem and suggest reasonable accommodations that they can take to resolve this. During all of this, keep a notebook with a listing of the grievances and the dates on which they took place. This will serve as evidence in the future, so be as specific and thorough as you can be.

If you are dissatisfied with the results of the complaint, turn to the local departments of the Equal Employment Opportunity Commission or the Department of Fair Employment and Housing and file a complaint with them. These departments should be listed in the telephone book. Both offices will ask you to fill out some paperwork to begin their investigation. This is where the notebook information will most likely help you. Another source of helpful information is your medical records. Depending on the caseload within these departments, it could take weeks or months for a resolution to your problem.

If you are still dissatisfied with the treatment of your complaint, you may want to contact an attorney. Be sure to use one who is fluent in employment law, particularly the latest case law surrounding the issue. There are a lot of charlatans out there. A knowledgeable attorney is one who is best equipped to pursue your claim through knowing and applying the law.

The FMLA

The second piece of law that is most likely on your side is the Family and Medical Leave Act (FMLA) of 1993. While many people link this law with maternity leave, it is also designed for those who are hospitalized for more than three days or those with conditions that require longer lengths of absence for treatment or recuperation of a serious illness.

Not all working people are covered by the FMLA. The provisions cover employees of the federal government, the state government and local governments, and schools. Employees in the private sector where the company has upwards of fifty employees in twenty or more workweeks are covered if the companies are engaged in industry or commerce. The fifty employees must be within a U.S. territory or the United States, and they must be within 75 miles of each other.

There are requirements of the employees as well. The provisions of the act cover a person if they have worked for a total of twelve months, during which time they have worked at least 1,250 hours (a forty-hour workweek over twelve months equals a total of 2,080 hours).

The law allows an employee who fits the requirements to have up to twelve weeks of leave to attend to the birth of a newborn or the adoption or foster care placement of a child. Additionally, an employee can use the time to recuperate from a serious health condition or to care for a seriously ill immediate family member. The time can be taken during one twelve-month period, the start of which is determined by the employer and can be the beginning of the leave, the end of the leave, or within a specified calendar period. The time can also be taken intermittently, meaning a regularly shortened workweek to schedule appointments or chunks of time taken now and then to deal with the matter.

Whether you are paid for the time or not is up to your employer. Some will cover portions of the time period, such as four weeks of maternity leave. Others will allow the use of accrued vacation days or similar time off and compensate accordingly for that time. You should check the terms of the matter in your employee handbook, if such a document exists.

In the case of IBD, you may want to check out the feasibility of using the FMLA in a few instances. If you require regular infusions of the drug Remicade, you may want to use the FMLA to schedule the time during regular workdays. For surgery, the FMLA is ideal since it allows for not only the immediate time in the hospital but also any time spent recuperating at home under a doctor's orders.

The FMLA provides protection of your job and benefits while you are on leave and when you return. While you are away, your employer must continue to supply you with health insurance benefits if these existed prior to your taking leave. Additionally, your original job or an equivalent job with similar pay and benefits must be available to you when you return. One exception to this is if you are one of the highest 10 percent salaried employees; in that case, a company can refuse to reinstate these employees, given proper notice is provided ahead of time. Under the law, employers can require the employee provide not only thirty-day notice of the intended leave but also medical certification of the illness, second or third medical opinions, and periodic updates once on leave.

The same types of steps that you take to enforce the ADA on your behalf can be taken here with one exception. The Wage and Hour Division of the U.S. Department of Labor is the investigator for complaints regarding this act; this division is listed in the front of most telephone books. Employment lawyers may also be consulted for violations of this law if civil redress is sought.

Realize that individual states have added certain restrictions on the two acts, thus strengthening the individual rights in many cases. Be sure to look at your own state's employment acts when considering action.

Other countries have adopted similar laws or have specific workplace laws that differ slightly. Be sure to seek counsel to determine your protection.

IN A SENTENCE:

There are laws to protect you and your job from discriminatory workplace practices.

DAY 4

living

Finding Solace and Support

THINK BACK to when you were a kid and had one of those inevitable spills. You know the ones, where your knee ended up being shaved by the sidewalk, and the injustice of it all—accompanied by the sharp pain—brought tears to your eyes. You probably hobbled back inside where your mother or some other loving, attentive adult cleaned you up, dressed your wounds, kissed away the tears, and sent you along again with a lollipop in your hand and a bright bandage on your leg.

Despite all the pain of the moment, those times were most likely pretty great, weren't they? When you were at your most sorrowful, you simply turned to others to calm, comfort, and reassure you. Within this first week of the disease, and for possibly weeks and months to come, you may yearn for that same source of comfort. You may not realize it but many of those same people and more are still there to hold your hand during this time of trial. In addition to family and friends, psychotherapists specializing in issues involving chronic illness or grief, and support groups for people with IBD most likely exist in your area. The Internet, filled with sites boasting Web message boards and chats, has support available for you at the click of your mouse.

When the World Trade Center was destroyed by terrorists, New York City residents, notorious for their brash attitudes and toughness, were bowled over with shock and sadness. Immediately, news reports spilled out about how people offered free water and juice on the sidewalks in front of their stores. Others opened their bathrooms to the public and still more took into their apartments some of the people who were left temporarily homeless by the blast. Everywhere, strangers reached out to pat each other on the back, offer a hug, or hold a hand; others who were farther away from Ground Zero gave their own blood and hundreds of millions of dollars to support the victims, their families, and the rescue work. That human touch was so very important to those suffering and grieving.

In many ways, finding your own support and solace at a time like this is the same. Something shocking and somewhat horrifying has happened to you, your own "Black Tuesday," to a lesser degree and scale. To go through it alone is unimaginable to most. We need others to sustain us in a time of grief and despair.

And, generally speaking, others are usually there to do just that. Options for people who are diagnosed with IBD include support groups, psychotherapists, and Internet chats and boards. You just have to know where to look.

Seeking help with a group

Free support groups are available through Crohn's & Colitis Foundation of America chapters (CCFA). Populated by groups of self-selected individuals with CD or UC, the groups usually meet once a month or every other month in a hospital setting or in space donated within an office building. Some support group leaders are psychologists and social workers who volunteer their time to lead the groups, but others are volunteers who are trained by the CCFA to handle the task. Bathrooms are never far and everyone understands if you have to suddenly excuse yourself.

Usually, the meetings begin with a question, a theme of the month, or an ice-breaker exercise, an interactive little game in which all participate to help initiate the conversation. Sometimes, there is an eight-week format that is followed. From the opening, generally, people can bring up their own issues or offer support to others. Participants share coping techniques and bits of humor that help them not only to get by, but also to reduce a little of the inherent stress in having a chronic illness. Occasionally, a professional such as a physician, a nurse practitioner, a dietitian, or a fitness expert will come to share a bit of IBD wisdom.

"Mutual support" is the catch phrase used to describe these meetings. The person who comes seeking help and assurance receives that from an individual who in turn obtains a boost in self-esteem from being able to help others. People who simply attend and don't contribute to the discussion are also beneficiaries, as they can see that they have plenty of company in their suffering with UC or CD.

While many people find a haven of sorts at these meetings, be aware that you may not be one of them. If talking openly to one person about the disease is hard, opening up to a group can be worse and because of this, it can be unbearably nerve-wracking to go. Finding trust is difficult for some at a meeting. Familiarity breeds trust, and people use these meetings sporadically as the need arises, so you may not see the same individuals time and again. In a similar vein, not everyone who attends the meetings is affected by the disease at the same level. People who attend may range from someone with mild symptoms who was just diagnosed to someone on **total parenteral nutrition (TPN)** with an **ostomy** who is constantly in pain.

Vickie first tried out the support groups when she was initially diagnosed. She and her cousin, both CD sufferers, attended together. Vickie was not doing well and was frightened about what the future would hold for her in terms of the disease.

"At that meeting, people were just telling their experiences about surgeries, TPN, et cetera. [What they had to say] scared me to death and I remember telling my cousin that I was not going to have any of the things they talked about," Vickie said.

Only you know whether a support group is for you. If you want to try one out, call your local CCFA chapter and ask for a listing of the times, dates, and locations of the upcoming support group meetings. Every chapter in the country has support groups, usually more than one. If you aren't sure how to locate your local chapter, check the phone book for the nearest location, or log on to the Web page for the national CCFA headquarters at www.ccfa.org. On the site, there are links to listings for all of the chapters arranged by state. Often, the information is listed on the chapter's individual page or can be had with a phone call.

Seeking help on an individual basis

Psychotherapists who deal in grief counseling or in the emotional issues that frequently surround chronic illness are another support option. These individuals—psychiatrists, psychologists, professional counselors, or clinical social workers—provide a good alternative if you aren't into support groups or are looking to explore some personal issues in an individualized setting.

The actual experience with a psychotherapist will vary from person to person as everyone has a different emotional makeup and issues to deal with. The session will usually take place in a small office and will last a pre-determined amount of time. There are a number of philosophies with which psychotherapists affiliate themselves, and the style of treatment will vary accordingly. Usually, however, the psychotherapist will ask a question and allow you to respond. Some psychotherapists will ask a lot of questions following the initial one while others will let you take it from there, filling in the details you find important. Certain psychotherapists will offer advice; others will allow you to come up with your own solutions through questions and discussion.

The price of psychotherapy is usually covered for a set period of time by your insurance. Therapy prices range widely and easily can exceed $100 an hour depending on the area of the country in which you live and the experience of the individual. If insurance covers the cost, a copay is most likely what you will have to shell out, the amount of which depends on the type of insurance coverage you have. Calling your insurance carrier and asking about your coverage will usually clear up any questions you might have about your coverage. If you are not covered for this service by your insurance or have no insurance, many psychotherapists offer sliding fee scales or payment plans.

If you are considering finding a psychotherapist, you might want to contact a professional association for psychotherapists; each one has its own guidelines and criteria for membership. All of the organizations below offer a referral service and can locate a psychotherapist in your area:

The National Registry of Certified Group Therapists
25 East 21st Street, 6th Floor
New York, New York 10010
www.agpa.org/group
(212) 477-2677; (877) 668-2472 (toll free)

The American Psychological Association Public Education Line
750 First Street, NE
Washington, DC 20002-4242
www.apa.org
(800) 374-2721

National Association of Social Workers
750 First Street, NE, Suite 700
Washington, DC 20002-4241
www.socialworkers.org
(202) 408-8600

American Counseling Association
5999 Stevenson Avenue
Alexandria, VA 22304
www.counseling.org
(800) 347-6647

American Psychiatric Association
1000 Wilson Boulevard, Suite 1825
Arlington, VA 22209-3901

There are a number of questions you should ask of a psychotherapist before agreeing to a therapy program. Perhaps the first should be to find out if the therapist is licensed by the state or local government. The licenses are critical as they show that the individual has gone through a certification process and is monitored for ethical practices. If you have questions about the person's licensing status, you can call the licensing governing body and ask if his or her license is current and when it expires. For most licensing agencies, you can also find out if the individual has had any grievances filed against him or her and, if so, how those grievances have been resolved.

The next questions can and should be answered by the psychotherapist before you agree to a treatment plan. First, find out how long they have been practicing. Certainly, newly minted psychotherapists are capable of handling their patients' issues, but some people feel more comfortable with a therapist who has been around for a little while. Then, find out what area the psychotherapist specializes in. If it is family therapy or marital therapy exclusively, this individual may not be for you unless you have issues to deal with in these areas as well. Next, find out how they operate by asking what kind of treatment plan they commonly use and why they find this to be effective. Finally, ask how long they expect the treatment will take. Some psychotherapists will say that this is something they can't judge until they have a better handle on the issues they are treating while others will give you a somewhat defined period of time. Beware of the psychotherapists who say that therapy is a lifelong endeavor; some psychotherapists see their clients as cash cows and keep people in therapy as long as they are footing the bill.

When I was diagnosed with CD, I coped on my own until the depression set in. I found myself crying over the simplest things and feeling overwhelmed a lot of the time. My boyfriend at the time—now my husband—was seeking his master's degree in psychology and suggested that I find someone to talk to about my feelings. Looking back, he was probably sick of my whining and crying. However, I followed his advice and lucked out in finding Audrey Kron, a psychologist with Crohn's disease who specializes in emotional issues surrounding chronic illness. I saw her weekly for about three or four months, talking almost exclusively about handling the implications of having a chronic illness. She truly helped me to see that I was more in control of a lot of the disease process than I thought I was. Without that time with her, I don't know how I would have gotten through my first year.

Seeking help on the Internet

Another option for support that more and more people are turning to is on the Internet. Web message boards, some with chat options available, are a popular place for people to hang out, to get to know each other, and to gripe all they want—for free. As you can imagine, this can be both good and bad.

The good part about these boards or online communities is that they let you know that you are not alone, that you are welcome and accepted, and that no symptom, no matter how gross or unspeakable, is too disgusting to be heard and discussed. The boards can be as anonymous as you need them to be, a plus for the timid or shy. People who wouldn't dream of telling a roomful of strangers that they have chronic bloody diarrhea or an itchy anus open up and let loose like never before. The sites are open 24 hours so when your prednisone is keeping you awake, you can communicate your suffering to fellow IBD sufferers. Many of the people who use these sites have a wealth of tips and information on the diseases, sharing breakthroughs in treatment options and medical advances faster than you can say "double blind study." And perhaps the greatest part is that they allow the users to reach out and voice their caring and concern for each other in a way that would otherwise be difficult, as many of the participants are separated physically by hundreds, at times thousands, of miles.

Just as the good part of the boards is that they are open to all, the bad part is that all come, including those who will urge you to dump the medications in place of unproven and, frankly, dangerous herbal therapies; those who are ill-informed but claim to be mavens; those who claim to know what the cure is and berate all those who don't follow them; and those who apparently have turned off their manners and good sense when they turned on the computers.

A lot of common sense is required to make this experience a good experience. Whatever information you receive on these boards has to be checked out through the use of medical studies, books, and, of course, your doctor. And never give out personal information such as your Social Security Number, credit card information, address, or telephone number to individuals on the Web.

IN A SENTENCE:

> *Psychological support is important and is available through a variety of sources.*

learning

How the Diseases Work

BY NOW, we have learned what the digestive system looks like, where it is located and how it works from the standpoint of the digestive process. It is important to have this base of knowledge as we prepare to understand how the diseases affect the gastrointestinal tract.

The inside view

If you were to take a piece of intestine and slice it open, you would find that it is a very interesting part filled with a diverse body of cells that each has its own function. Starting from the innermost surface to the outer, the cells are aligned to absorb nutrients, fight invaders, transmit nerve responses, transport oxygen and red blood cells, and move the contents of the intestines through.

The innermost layer is the mucosa, a thin layer of cells that surrounds the hollow part of the intestines, the space in which is called the **lumen.** A principal part of this is the **epithelium,** which is made up of epithelial cells known as villi and microvilli. These tiny finger and oak-leaf like projections in the intestines are essential to the human body as they help to regulate the

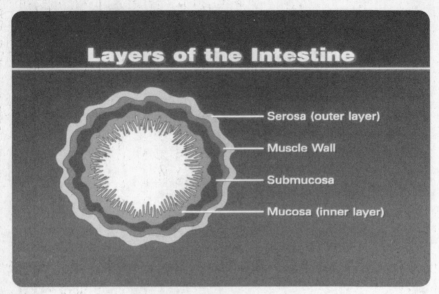

Different cells and layers play a part in digestion.

©*Crohn's & Colitis Foundation of America (CCFA). Reprinted with permission of CCFA.*

absorption of not only essential nutrients but also water, hundreds of ounces of which pass through us each day. Epithelial cells are found in the intestines and also in the skin, the breast, and a number of other locations in the body.

Stationed beneath the epithelium are areas where new epithelial cells are being born and nurtured. Should the epithelium be damaged, these areas, known as crypts, spring into action and repair the epithelium, restoring it to its former strength and capability within hours. In spaces around and in between the crypts lie an army of immune cells that make up the mucosa and underlying submucosa; these cells perform the task of protecting the body from invading bacteria that are ingested. These cells—including eosinopils, neutrophils, mast cells, lymphocytes, and macrophages—respond to the invaders by eating them or attaching antibodies to them to destroy them or inhibit their attempt to permeate the bowel wall. These cells are key to IBD, and we will learn more about them in the following sections.

Next in line is the complex system of nerve cells and muscle cells that work together called the **muscularis.** The nerve cells receive information from neurotransmitters and hormones and forward this information through a series of connections known as the enteric nervous system to the brain. This intricate network helps to regulate peristalsis by interpreting neurotransmitters and hormones and then triggering the muscles to squeeze. The two layers of muscles, the circular muscles and the longitudinal muscles, work together to move the intestinal contents through. The circular muscles contract one after another in a wavelike fashion while the longitudinal muscles shorten and lengthen, like the movement a worm makes to move. Whatever the villi and microvilli don't absorb, these muscles push further down.

Finally, the serosa is the outer layer of the intestines, a protective lining of sorts. The serosa acts to keep possible invaders from entering the peritoneum, the cavity in which the intestines reside. If the bacteria do enter the peritoneum, it can cause a potentially deadly infection called **peritonitis.**

The inflammatory process

In CD and UC, an inflammatory process takes place. As stated before, UC causes the inflammation to take place at the mucosal level in the colon only, while CD is marked by inflammation that pierces the mucosa, the muscularis and, occasionally, the serosa.

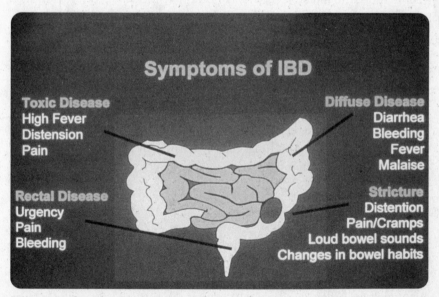

Different symptoms point to varying disease activity.
©*Crohn's & Colitis Foundation of America (CCFA). Reprinted with permission of CCFA*

Sometimes the epithelium barrier is not enough to stave off invading bacteria that creep in between spaces called tight junctions. Permeating the barrier, the invaders cause the immune cells to gather at the site to destroy them. This is not to say that a bacterial, parasitic, or viral invader is the cause of IBD. Rather, this is the response that is mounted by the immune system. It may be that the cause for the reaction is the immune cells misreading normal bacteria as invaders and then launching a sustained attack.

Chemical signals contained within the immune cells are released in an inflammatory response. At the same time, tiny blood vessels dilate, delivering more red blood cells to the site. Fluid also floods the area, causing swelling that is known as **edema**. The epithelium can erode at the site and allow more immune cells to traverse the epithelial barrier, which results in ulcerations and deep, crevicelike formations. In CD, the inflammation burrows through, at times all the way through the serosa. When the serosa is pierced, immune cells work to quickly surround the infection, causing an abscess to form. The contents of the abscess are the rapidly multiplying and dying bacteria.

As the inflammation builds and damages the mucosa, the nerve system is alerted to the inflammation. In response, it can cause the muscles to contract to move the intestinal contents faster over the injured area, resulting in muscle spasms in some. The mucosa, busy with and hampered by the inflammation, forgo absorbing the water, bile salts, and nutrients. As the inflammation subsides, scar tissue can be left on the mucosa, leaving areas where epithelial cells do not exist anymore.

Again, no one is exactly sure what causes the inflammation in the first place. It could be an immune system gone haywire, a logical reaction to a bacterial breach of the epithelium, a tiny microbe that has taken up residence, or maybe a genetic fluke that is causing all of this. The potential causes will be more thoroughly examined in Day 7.

The causes of the symptoms

It can be hard to believe that something that is happening so microscopically on the cellular level can have such a major impact on the way we feel, but it is true. Fever, abdominal pain, weight loss, diarrhea, and anemia are all ways that our body tells us that the action at the cellular level is out of whack, especially in the case of IBD.

With fever, the body's internal temperature rises, a sign of activity in IBD that can be an indication of an inflammatory response or a bacterial infection. In the inflammatory response, certain immune cells are involved in a complex physiological chain of events that cause a pyrogenic (*pyro* meaning fire) response, raising the temperature and metabolism of the body. A bacterial infection is the result of an abscess, as happens in CD, or can happen in UC when the bacteria-laden contents of the colon spill into the peritoneum as a result of a dangerous happenstance called **toxic megacolon.** The immune response causes the temperature to escalate to a high level rapidly, and often produces chills as well.

Abdominal pain can be the result of several disease activities. The swelling at the site of the inflammation can cause a cramping pain not too dissimilar from that skinned knee suffered at the beginning of the chapter. During a physical exam of the abdomen, a doctor can feel the inflammatory mass and may press down on it to see if it hurts. When the swelling and scar tissue become too much and block the intestines, the wavelike squeezing pain occurs as the intestines attempt to force their contents through a tiny opening. This is known as a partial or complete obstruction and the pain has been known to be harder than the labor associated with childbirth. The abdominal pain that is knifelike, sharp, and very sensitive to touch is usually related to an abscess. Finally, a cramping pain often accompanies digestion or evacuation of the bowels. This may be the result of the muscle layers being burrowed through by the disease process or an underlying motility disorder.

Diarrhea is the result of water and bile salts that are not properly absorbed during the digestive process. When the epithelial cells are not able to work properly due to inflammatory response, the water is not able to be absorbed. The colon has more water to contend with, leaving the fecal matter less formed or entirely liquid. More contractions by the intestinal muscle lead to more trips to the toilet.

Weight loss can be both a mental response as well as a physiological response to the disease process. It is not unreasonable for individuals with fever or severe abdominal pain to lose their appetite nor is it hard to understand why the person who makes twenty to thirty trips to the bathroom in a day doesn't want to add any food to their system that will meet a similar quick transit time, the length of time food takes to go from the mouth to the anus. Nor is it difficult to understand that a damaged gut is less able to absorb from food the items the body needs to sustain normal activity. Often times a quick transit time will leave some foods undigested and therefore unabsorbed.

Fatigue as well as anemia are really the result of all of the different symptoms. Any one of the symptoms can leave an individual with a tired, worn out feeling, but can really take the toll on the person's strength when endured in combination for days or weeks. Anemia, the presence of too few red blood cells (erythrocytes), is often the result of blood loss in IBD. As the intestinal layers become more inflamed, the dilation of the blood vessels allows for more blood to be released, often through ulceration. The greater or more sustained the blood loss, the more severe the anemia. With fewer red blood cells to cart oxygen around the body, the feeling of fatigue becomes more prevalent. Other symptoms associated with anemia include pale looking skin, weakness, lightheadedness, and an increased susceptibility to changes in temperature.

IN A SENTENCE:

> *In the intestine's complex environment, even microscopic inflammatory changes can cause effects felt throughout the body.*

Assembling Your Health Care Team

"NO MAN is an island, entire of itself; every man is a piece of the continent, a part of the main," John Donne once wrote, and hardly has that been more true than with the treatment of IBD. To get through this disease, you need to be able to rely on the help, expertise, and advice of health care professionals such as your primary care physician (PCP), your gastroenterologist, your **colorectal surgeon,** and your nutritionist or registered dietitian. These individuals will either sink or save you, which is why it is so critically important for you to carefully choose these individuals to be a part of your health care team.

Notice the word "team" in the last sentence. This means that you are still an active participant. At no time in the treatment of your disease should you hand the reins over to others to make your decisions. Rather, try to look at these people as your support staff or teammates, ones who will help you to wage the battle.

In fact, your decision making begins this very minute. As you read this today, take stock of who is on this team. Figure out who you want to keep and who you want to replace. Try to list what your options are. Is your gastroenterologist really one who is right for you or should you search for another one? Does your nutritionist truly have a familiarity with IBD or is that person better suited to treat heart patients? Is your surgeon kind and compassionate or a mini-dictator without a country but with you as his or her constituent?

There are many reasons that you shouldn't necessarily settle for the health care provider for whom you are given a referral. It is not that this individual isn't the best person out there; plenty of us get lucky on this first shot. But how will you know if you don't ask the questions?

As consumers, we ask questions about just about every major decision that we make in our lives. If you were going to put an addition onto your dwelling, you would call a few builders, check out their quotes, and demand to see examples of their work before you signed on the dotted line. If you were going to an expensive restaurant, you would at least read a review or get a recommendation from a friend before venturing out. And that car you were considering locking into a three-year lease with? You'd be sure to take it for a test drive or kick the tires.

But when it comes to doctors and other health care providers, most of us are willing to take whoever comes along. We know almost nothing about where they went to school, how much experience they have, or what their philosophy regarding the treatment of IBD is, and yet we trust them implicitly with our care and follow their instructions for medication or surgery. After all, they wouldn't let just anyone into medical schools, much less wear the white coat, would they?

Remember, there are huge benefits to having a trusting relationship with your health care provider. Studies have shown that if you trust your doctor and believe in the treatment she or he prescribes, you will most likely be compliant, a term that means you follow their instructions for medical care. So taking your time and doing your homework before choosing your PCP, gastroenterologist, surgeon, and nutritionist or registered dietitian will pay off for you in the end.

Again, I am not suggesting that you go out and kick your doctor or take your nutritionist for a test drive. Rather, I suggest carefully researching and interviewing your health care providers before signing up with them for the long haul. And I do mean long haul. Until a cure is found, consider CD incurable and UC curable only through the loss of the lower GI tract. In light of this, we are talking about a long-term commitment.

The first steps

To first locate a health care provider, it is helpful to try to cull recommendations from people you know and trust. Ask them who they use and why they use them. Ask for specific examples of a nutritionist's knowledge or of a doctor's compassion. And if they can't recommend the person, ask for specific examples of that, too. If no one you know uses a gastroenterologist, for example, a call to your local CCFA chapter may be helpful. The chapters maintain a physician membership roster that is available to the public and, more importantly, there are individuals within the chapter who can vouch for certain health care providers.

Another way of gathering names of health care providers is to contact some of the professional organizations that represent them. Many of these organizations have professional requirements that the individual must achieve on an ongoing basis; the organizations also offer education and support to their membership. Nearly all of these organizations have a health care provider locator system, many of which are easily accessible online (www.eatright.org for registered dietitians, www.gastro.org for gastroenterologists, www.abcrs.org for colorectal surgeons, www.aafp.org for family physicians, www.ama-assn.org for all medical doctors, www.aap.org for pediatricians).

Once you have the names and telephone numbers of prospective health care providers, you may want to call the office and ask the receptionist the following questions:

○ Find out which health care plans are accepted in the office. Paying for these services out of pocket can be very expensive, even with sliding scales that are sometimes offered.

○ In the case of doctors, find out with which hospital that individual is affiliated. If you simply must use Hospital X due to strong personal preference and Dr. Y is not affiliated with that hospital, it is not the end of the world, as some hospitals honor visiting doctor privileges.

○ Ask whether or not the person is accepting any new patients. Some health care providers are so overbooked that they simply can't take on another patient. If that is the case, keep the individual's name handy for future reference.

○ Discuss logistics. Dr. A may be the best, most knowledgeable doctor on the face of the earth with an opening for you but if you have to drive five hours to see her, you can bet you won't feel comfortable calling with seemingly minor issues.

Next, check out the health care providers with a few agencies that monitor the doctors. A quick phone call or website visit to your state's Board of Medicine or similar licensing and regulation body will provide you with information such as whether or not the person is licensed to practice medicine. Depending on the state, these regulatory bodies can also tell you if there has been any disciplinary action against the individual or if there have been complaints filed against him or her. Don't think that you are overdoing it by seeking out this information; you may save yourself some heartache by doing so now rather than finding out later.

Another place to look for information is with the medical boards that certify these individuals. Board certification is a process by which the individual health care provider has to complete requisite education and training programs and must be tested extensively about their knowledge in the area in which they practice every 6 to 10 years. This assures the certifying board that the individual who claims membership is up on the advances in the field and is competent to practice. The American Medical Association (www.ama-assn.org) has a function on its Web site that allows for patients to seek information on the doctors such as training and board certification. In the United States, the American Board of Medical Specialties hosts a Web site (www.abms.org) that lists all twenty-four boards recognized in the country. The site also hosts a search engine that allows you to plug in the name of the doctor to find out whether or not that individual is board certified. For gastroenterology, there is currently not a separate board entity as there is with colorectal surgeons; however, GIs are certified with the American Board of Internal Medicine, with subspecialty certification in gastroenterology.

After you have narrowed your selection, set up an appointment to interview the health care provider. Depending on the individual, you may have to pay for the time out of pocket but it is worth it to do so. Jot down all of the questions you have ahead of time in a notebook, bring a pen, and be prepared to take notes. Treat this time like a job interview. It is in many ways, after all. You will be giving this person the task of taking care of your medical, surgical, or nutritional needs.

The following are some of the specialties you may need in health care providers, and there is a list of questions on page 60 that you might want to ask them.

The primary care physician

In recent years, the term "primary care physician" has come to mean just about anyone in any specialty. In fact, during a recent conference, one neurosurgeon introduced himself to the crowd as a "primary care neurosurgeon." As ludicrous as that seems, it is because of a movement by the health maintenance organizations (HMOs) to restrict access to specialists by requiring referrals from health care providers who are designated as PCPs. These gatekeepers of the medical system seem to have their hands on the reins of the medical establishment, providing work through referrals to the doctors as they directed patients at will.

Without getting into the medical history or politics of the movement, it is important to know what a PCP is and what they do. A PCP is a doctor who takes care of ailments of the entire body, from healing sore throats to treating nasty foot fungus. These doctors are educated in an undergraduate program at the college level, followed by four years in medical school, and three to seven years in training periods called internships and residencies. Pediatricians, doctors who specialize in the care of children and young adults, are PCPs, as are their adult medicine counterparts, internists. Family medical specialists care for individuals, regardless of age, sex, or medical concern.

When these physicians encounter a difficult disease to treat, they will refer the patient to another doctor who specializes in the body part that is affected. Often times, a PCP is the physician who diagnoses the condition. That is because the PCP is usually the one we see when the symptoms first appear. Your choice of a PCP is important in the treatment of your IBD; the more that individual knows about your condition, the better the treatment you will receive. Be sure that this individual is aware of the medications you can and can't take, and has at least a general knowledge of the condition.

The gastroenterologist

A gastroenterologist, or GI, is a specialist who likely went through four years of undergraduate education at the college level, four years of medical school, three years of an internship (most likely in internal medicine), and one to three more years of training in the subspecialty. Some of these doctors also have more specific training in hepatology—the study of the liver and its functions—because the liver has a key role in digestion.

The specialty of gastroenterology covers the entire digestive tract including the esophagus, the stomach, the small intestines, the gallbladder, the pancreas, the liver, the large intestine, the rectum, and the anus. Outside of the treatment of IBD, the diseases they treat include, but are not limited to, all of the hepatitis viruses, gallbladder disease, diverticulosis, **irritable bowel syndrome**, celiac disease, helicobacter pylori infections (ulcers), and genetic polyp disease. Some specialize in just one of the diseases, often doing research on the disease, while others treat the whole spectrum.

Because of their internal medicine background, a gastroenterologist may serve as your PCP. If you choose to have separate doctors for these purposes, the gastroenterologist should be able to relate well with your PCP as well as your surgeon, if there is a need for one. The GI may also be a great referral source for a nutritionist or registered dietitian, as they often work with these professionals.

The colorectal surgeon

A colorectal surgeon is someone who has likely gone through four years of undergraduate education at the college level, four years of medical school, five years of training in general surgery, and another year of training in the specialized field.

Generally, these individuals do the vast majority of their work in the stomach, small intestines, the colon, rectum, anal canal, and perianal area, but they also do most of their training in general surgery and thus can treat many areas of the body. Some of the diseases they treat include colon cancer, polyps, diverticulitis, hemorrhoids, and **fissures.** Colorectal surgeons are also trained in the medical treatment of the diseases they treat surgically. Like gastroenterologists, some of these surgeons have sub-subspecialties, meaning they are known as a maven in just one of the diseases like a colon cancer specialist or an IBD specialist.

If experience is key anywhere in dealing with these illnesses, it is in the field of surgery. You may not feel comfortable having an individual perform your subtotal **colectomy** if you are only this surgeon's fifth patient to go through with it.

The nutritionist or registered dietitian

The field of nutrition in IBD has been a hotbed of controversy pretty much since the diseases were discovered. But no one debates the importance of having a good nutrition program in place, if for no other reason to make sure that the basic nutrients, vitamins, and minerals are in the diet. A nutrition specialist will also be able to tell you which foods to eliminate from the diet in order to avoid more diarrhea.

A nutritionist is a person who uses the science of nutrition to improve health. There is no accreditation process for a nutritionist as there is for a registered dietitian (RD) through the American Dietetic Association. To attain accreditation, a RD must have completed an accredited four-year degree program that is approved by the ADA. (A personal note: Don't be quick to dismiss the nutritionist, but be sure to examine their credentials. The individual I receive nutrition advice from is an internationally known fitness expert and former Mr. Universe who happens to have Crohn's disease. He is not an RD, but he has consistently given me better nutrition advice than the RD I consulted with who knew little about the disease, insisting that I choose foods to "boost" my immune system when I was trying to suppress it medically, and admonishing me for not eating more roughage when I had a stricture.) The course work includes biochemistry, biology, and diet therapy, and the candidates have to pass a national exam administered by the ADA. If it is important to you, be sure to ask where the individual received training and education as well as what type of certification they hold.

A nutritionist or RD will examine your current diet and recommend a diet plan for you to ensure optimum health. They may also recommend supplements such as calcium, folic acid, and vitamin E. You may find that you prefer one who has had exposure to IBD and is knowledgeable about the side effects of treatments. Because of this, you may want to ask the people at your CCFA chapter for suggestions or the doctors with whom you are working; be sure to also ask this question of them in the interview. Also query them on their knowledge of the effects of medical and surgical treatment on absorption of nutrients.

One thing to remember in particular when choosing a nutritional specialist is that insurance does not always cover the expense. Call your benefits representative to see if the visit is covered. Most likely, you will meet with your nutritionist or RD for a limited amount of time so handling the out of pocket costs probably won't be a major hardship. Even so, find out how many visits are required before committing to treatment.

Dumping your doctor

Occasionally, you may find that your doctor's services are not able to meet your needs or achieve good results. Or perhaps you will have a huge, messy disagreement about the way the (insert your description here) handles your case. If you are on either end of the spectrum, or anywhere in between, you have come to the great conundrum that some people with IBD face at times: how to dump the doctor without screwing yourself?

Sometimes when you can control the situation, it is better to try to work out the differences. If you feel you have been mistreated in some way or the lines of communication are down, discuss this at your next appointment. If you feel that the doctor has made an unnecessary change in your medication, call him or her and take up the topic concisely. But if you can't get past the issue, can't resolve the situation, or never feel like you are being heard, it might be best to find another physician to treat you.

Some things you can't change, like a shift in your insurance or a move on either party's part. The move may be an insurmountable issue unless you are willing and able to travel the distance. If you have an insurance issue that forces the switch, first see if there are alternatives or remedies that you can pursue before making the switch.

When the change is inevitable, be upfront about it, but be as kind and as calm as you possibly can be, even if it literally means biting your tongue in tense situations. As much as you may like to tell the health care provider what you think about his or her bedside manner, don't; you will likely be burning a bridge you may have to cross yet again. If you liked your doctor but have to change, this won't be difficult. Ask the doctor to send copies of all of your medical records to your next doctor. Doctor Number Two will probably request that information when you have your initial consultation. Still, it may cushion any perceived blow if Doctor Number One knows about the impending transition ahead of time. Ask Doctor Number One to consult with Doctor Number Two to discuss your case.

IN A SENTENCE:

Be a smart consumer when choosing a health care team.

Questions for the doctor

YOU are at the first meeting with your doctor. You have shaken his or her hand and are now sitting across from each other. Now is the time to begin asking the questions of the doctor. But what to ask?

Below is a list of general questions you can ask your PCP, your GI, and your colorectal surgeon, followed by more specialized questions you might want to ask the GI and the surgeon if you choose to have one of these doctors as your primary IBD doctor. Be selective in asking the questions, however; asking them all of the questions may make your physician run for the hills rather than accept you as a patient. I cannot stress how important it is during this interview to try to get a feel for not only the doctor's competence, but also his or her compassion. That said, don't let your feelings go with only your first impression; only time and your experience with the physician will allow you to form a complete opinion about these qualities.

One final note: I tend to ask the first question on the first list entirely for personal reasons. It is a joy to work with individuals who are passionate about what they do, not biding their years until retirement or in it for the money.

1. Why did you choose the field in which you practice?
   Do you like what you do?
2. How much experience do you have with UC or CD?
3. How many patients do you currently have who have IBD?
4. How would you work with the other doctors who are treating me?
5. What would the protocol be for me to follow should I have a fever or another symptom that could be either my IBD or something entirely different?
6. What would the protocol be for hospitalization be if it is for my disease?
7. Do you have experience with the latest treatments for IBD?

For the GI and surgeon, more specific questions that would be appropriate to ask include the following:

1. What can I expect treatment to be in mild, moderate, and severe cases?
2. Are there any medications or treatments that you avoid? Why?
3. What role do you believe nutrition should play?

4. For what reasons are tests scheduled? How often will I have colonoscopies?

5. How many endoscopic procedures have you performed? What is the complication rate you have experienced? What kinds of complications have you experienced?

6. If I have an emergency situation arise such as an abscess, what is the protocol that I should follow to get in touch with you?

7. Under what other circumstances should I call you? Are there others who would take your calls if you were not available? Do they have similar experience?

8. What is your preference in treating pain caused by the disease?

9. Should I have to have surgery, what types of pain management techniques do you employ? How many of each surgical procedure have you performed on people with IBD? What is your fatality rate? What happened in those circumstances?

10. Will you provide me with information about the disease? Can I bring in information that I find and discuss it with you?

11. How do you feel about alternative medicine and treatments?

learning

The Intestinal Complications of IBD

INTESTINAL COMPLICATIONS of CD and UC are certainly not everyday occurrences in IBD patients, even if you are experiencing one right now. Abscesses, fistulas, obstructions, toxic megacolon, **perforations**, and **fulminant colitis** may never be experienced by an individual with the disease. However, it is very important to understand what the complications are, what they feel like, and how they are diagnosed and treated in case one should happen along.

Abscesses and Fistulas

Much more common in CD, the formation of these two complications begins with a breach in the mucosa, caused by uncontrolled inflammation. Bacteria present in the intestines take up residence in the little hole in the intestinal wall, while a variety of white cells set upon them in an immune system attack. As the bacterial and immune cells do battle, more bacteria continue to empty into a pocket that begins to form, adding to some of the immune and bacterial cells that have perished. The mess of living and dead cells begin to bulge outward, pressing forward and through the muscularis and the serosa at times.

The abscessed mass can press up against another organ such as the bladder, can push outward to the skin, or can bear down on another segment of intestines. As it does so, it can radiate a knifelike, sharp pain when touched. To the touch, the surface can be hot and hard and the abscess is full of a goopy pus, colored yellow to green, that is slowly breaking through the adjacent organ, skin, or intestinal loop that it touches. The abscess can also cause fever with chills and fatigue.

If it is difficult to imagine, it might help to think of the abscess like a water balloon. As a trickle of water enters the balloon, the water is easily contained. As the balloon fills with water, the sides stretch taut to contain the water. And as with a water balloon, you don't want it to burst and the contents to spill all over the place. In this case, the consequences of spilled bacteria in the peritoneum can be a potentially deadly infection.

Abscesses can be diagnosed in different ways but are commonly found using an ultrasound or CT scan or blood tests which can reveal an elevated white cell count signaling potential infection. These noninvasive tests don't hurt and are quickly performed. When the abscess is between the intestines and the skin, the abscess can be palpitated by the physician or even seen at times. When visible, an abscess looks like a boil. To treat the abscess, a physician can lance the abscess using a scalpel or needle; depending on the size and location of an abscess, surgery may be required. To clear up the remaining pus, antibiotics like ciprofloxacin hydrochloride (Cipro), and metronidazole (**Flagyl**) usually are prescribed; other antibiotics include omnipen (ampicillin) and gentamycin.

A common frustration in treating abscesses that many IBD patients experience is that the space formed by the abscess remains after the pus is cleared up can easily refill with bacteria, repeating the whole scenario over and over. This situation is possible because the entrance to the abscess does not always close. When this is the case and the area is easily accessible to the doctor, the abscess is drained, cleaned, and packed with sterile surgical gauze that is changed frequently. The hope is that the opening of the abscess will heal. At times, the area may be resected or strictureplasty may be performed to eliminate the abscess. For more on surgical procedures, see Months 2 and 3.

CROHN'S DISEASE AND ULCERATIVE COLITIS

When the abscess pushes through another organ, the skin, or another segment of intestine, it can burst, thus relieving the painful pressure. The pus will then trickle out and can clear up with the aid of the antibiotics previously mentioned. The hope, of course, is that both the entrance and the exit points of the pus will heal and bowel activity will return to normal, but that doesn't always happen. When it doesn't, a fistula is born. A fistula is like a little hallway between the diseased intestine and its destination, be it the organ, the skin, or the other bowel segment.

Like abscesses, fistulas can be diagnosed on sight as fecal matter or bowel contents escape through abnormal openings. Depending on the location of a fistula, barium X-rays such as a small bowel series or a barium enema can also pinpoint the location of a fistula, as the barium appears to take an alternate path away from the intestines when it leaks into the fistula opening.

Fistulas aren't always a bad thing, especially when they are between two segments of closely located small bowel segments (enteroenteral). In fact, you may not know they exist within you. The bowel contents simply drain from one spot to another. Even when they are located between the rectum or anus and the skin (rectocutaneous or anocutaneous) or the rectum and the vagina (rectovaginal), the fistula may end up being a minor annoyance, causing one to simply wipe up occasional stray fecal matter or mucous.

However, they can become dangerous. For example, a fistula that allows the contents of the bowel to empty into the bladder can cause a serious bladder infection. A sign of such a fistula would be fecal matter that passes into the urine stream, urine that has the appearance of tomato soup, or air passing through the urinary opening. Another complication occurs when the fistula opens to the skin (enterocutaneous). Here, bacteria not only passes out of the intestine but the intestine is also exposed to bacteria from the outside world.

Treating a fistula is not a simple equation whereby patient A takes medicine B, and undergoes surgery C to result in cure D. There are a number of factors to consider, even within a single patient. Antiobiotics [metronidazole (Flagyl) and ciprofloxacin (Cipro)], corticosteroids [prednisone, prednisolone, and budesonide (Entocort)] immunosuppressives [6-mercaputopurine (Purinethol), azathioprine (Imuran, Azasan), cyclosporine (Sandimmune, Neoral), tacrolimus (Prograf), and methotrexate (Rheumatrex, MTX)], and biologics [infliximab (Remicade)] are all used with varying degrees of success in treating fistulas. Because of that, doctors can choose to start with antibiotics in one patient, move to steroids and immunosuppressives, and be done with it, while another patient may already be on immunosuppressives and may require a round of the biologic drug infliximab (Remicade), and still another may require surgical intervention. If the medications don't work or aren't well tolerated, a few surgical options are available, such as resection of the segment of the intestine to which the fistula is connected and the removal of the fistula itself. For those fistulas in close proximity to the rectum and anus, a flap can be cut in the mucosa that is brought down to cover the opening of the fistula, causing the fistula to dry up. A temporary **colostomy** also can be performed to divert waste from the area, also allowing the fistula to heal; the colostomy is then reversed at a later date. Another surgical option involves passing a wire through the fistula to the opening in the bowel wall and debriding or removing dead skin around the wound at the opening of the fistula, allowing the opening to scar over and heal closed.

Toxic megacolon, fulminant colitis, and toxic colitis

A potentially deadly complication requiring hospitalization and possibly surgery, toxic megacolon is more common among UC patients than CD patients. Fortunately, it affects the entire IBD population only in small percentages.

This complication generally begins with an onset of serious symptoms such as severe abdominal pain, fever, dehydration, and rapid heartbeat. A patient will appear pale and clammy, feel weak and faint, and be in great pain. In blood tests, usually there is an increase in white blood cells and platelets and a decrease in hemoglobin and albumin, leaving the patient to feel the effects of anemia; sodium and potassium levels may also be markedly low. In UC patients, this condition is known as fulminant colitis and has been known to happen in fewer than 10 percent of patients. Usually, the condition happens in UC patients in whom medical treatment has failed or to a lesser degree in patients in whom a UC diagnosis was recently made. In CD patients, the condition is called toxic colitis and is rare.

The first approach to managing toxic colitis and fulminant colitis is to attempt to return the patient to normal blood and electrolyte levels through blood transfusions and intravenous infusions of potassium and sodium. Patients may also receive intravenous steroids and **Cyclosporine,** a rapidly acting immunosuppressant. To relieve the built-up pressure caused by swallowed air, the doctor may order that a **nasogastric tube** be placed up the patient's nose, down the throat, and into the stomach to suction off the excessive air, and digestive secretions such as bile. Doctors usually prescribe bowel rest and avoid prescribing anticholinergic, narcotic, and antidiarrhea drugs, as they tend to slow the activity of the colon.

During the next twenty-four to forty-eight hours, several X-rays may be taken of the abdomen to check the dilation of the colon, a sign that the condition has progressed. Most likely no colonoscopy or barium X-ray will be performed as both of these carry risks of perforation of the colon. However a sigmoidoscopy may be done to make sure that the diagnosis is colitis. A consultation with a surgeon may also take place because the fear is that the toxic colitis or fulminant colitis will progress to the most dangerous complication in IBD, toxic megacolon.

Toxic megacolon occurs when the muscles of the colon become paralyzed, allowing the gases of the bacteria in the colon to multiply. With no muscular action to shove the gases out of the colon, the gases collect and their growing volume pushes upon the now flaccid muscles. The colon then becomes like a balloon, growing larger and threatening perforation. The transverse colon is usually the first segment of the colon to show the change but every area of the colon can be affected.

Surgery is really the only option during this dire phase, as perforation of the colon will almost assuredly lead to peritonitis, a potentially lethal infection that occurs when intestinal contents spill into the peritoneum during a perforation. In most cases, the colon must be surgically removed while care is taken to prevent infection. For more information on surgical options, see Months 2 and 3.

Perforation

In both CD and UC, the risk of perforation exists, though usually as a result of another complication of the disease. With UC, the perforation is a risk with toxic megacolon, as mentioned above, while the perforation can occur in CD with the presence of an abscess or fistula.

In either case, the patient experiences sudden, severe abdominal pain that is made worse with movement. A sudden high fever and chills usually follow. An elevated white blood cell count indicates a bacterial infection. As discussed above, the overflow of the contents of the intestine into the peritoneum can lead to peritonitis, a potentially lethal infection of the abdominal cavity. Because of this danger, immediate surgery is usually called for to remove the colon or to resect the affected area. Antibiotics can be taken to battle the possible bacterial infection.

Strictures, obstructions, and adhesions

Inflammation is a cause for a concern not only for the way it makes the patient feel, but also for the danger it presents in terms of the formation of strangling adhesions and **strictures** that can lead to obstructions.

Strictures happen most often in CD, in particular in the terminal ileum. (In UC, a stricture may be the result of the formation of colon cancer. See Month 5 for more information.) In part, strictures happen here most often because this area is the most common location for CD but also because this segment gradually narrows until it reaches the ileocecal valve. When inflammation or the resultant scar tissue crowd this area, the opening through which food and air can pass becomes smaller and smaller. One way to visualize this is to imagine a six-lane highway suddenly narrowed to one lane for the purpose of an accident or construction. Just as an angry snarl of cars with an angrier mass of drivers would result on that highway, so too does a backup of food and air accumulate with a partial or complete obstruction in the intestines.

To remedy this, the body attempts to shove the backed up food and air through the tiny opening using waves of peristalsis. These attempts not only produce loud sounds (noisy peristalsis) but also intensely squeezing pain, nausea, and vomiting. The abdomen can become uncomfortably distended and walking in an upright position may seem impossible. The episode can last a half an hour to several hours.

To diagnose an obstruction, X-rays of the abdomen are ordered. In a full obstruction, no evidence of stool or air will have passed on the other side of the affected area, while a partial obstruction will allow small amounts through. In treating an obstruction, time is the greatest ally as many obstructions will resolve themselves. A narcotic pain reliever such as morphine, Demerol, or Dilaudid may help take the edge off the pain but won't entirely relieve it. A nasogastric tube can help to reduce the buildup of swallowed air and digestive secretions. When the patient is doing better, clear liquids and semi-liquids like Jell-O, chicken broth, and apple juice are given. If that food is tolerated well, softer foods can be added to the diet slowly. Eventually, the patient may have to adopt a low fiber diet to reduce the chance of recurrence.

To prevent a further obstruction, a doctor may prescribe more anti-inflammatory medication like prednisone or **budesonide** (**Entocort**) to lessen any inflammation that may be causing the obstruction. If scar tissue is the cause of the obstruction, a surgical resection may be the only option, as there is no medication available to treat scar tissue. Adhesions, scar tissue on the outside of the intestine that is usually the result of surgery or severe disease, can also cause the obstruction by wrapping around the intestines, thus restricting the flow of the intestinal contents. These would have to be surgically cut away.

Massive hemorrhage

A rare occurrence in both CD and UC, massive hemorrhage causes a great loss of blood over a short period of time, minutes, or hours instead of days or weeks. In UC, the patient is usually very ill and the occurrence can be a sign of toxic colitis. For CD patients, massive hemorrhage can happen when the person is very ill or relatively well, and can happen when an errant ulceration drills its way into a blood vessel in the colon.

The patient who is experiencing a major loss of blood through hemorrhage will most likely feel dizzy, faint, and cold. When they go to the bathroom, they will likely feel a lot of liquid escaping and see the toilet bowl filled with blood, so much so that other toilet bowl contents are obscured from sight. A doctor may find that the patient has low blood pressure but a rapid pulse, or that their hemoglobin and albumin are low on a blood test.

Medically, a hemorrhage can be treated by infusing the patient with blood products to promote clotting. Once the patient is more stable, transfusions of blood can help to restore blood levels or injections of a synthetic hormone called epogen can help to prompt the body to produce more red blood cells. At times, the hemorrhage resolves itself and no treatment is needed.

Surgery, however, may be required, and may call for the removal of the colon or the segment of diseased intestines to prevent a possibly fatal recurrence.

IN A SENTENCE:

> *Intestinal complications for CD and UC range from common to rare, but all can be dangerous.*

When to Call the Doctor

BY NOW, you probably realize from what you have learned that having IBD means living with a little uncertainty. Things may be going great for months on end when suddenly you begin to feel yucky. Maybe a fever hits and no cold or flu symptoms follow. Possibly you log more time in the bathroom during numerous trips. Or perhaps you have symptoms of serious intestinal complications discussed in Day 5.

Whatever the case, it is smart to take your concerns to your doctor instead of trying to handle the situation yourself. Knowing what to do in such a case, be it a minor annoyance or a major emergency, will help you to feel more confident and in control in any situation.

Notable symptoms

Not all IBD symptoms warrant a call to the doctor. A few extra trips to the bathroom in a day or a bit of blood noticed while wiping are generally to be expected, but abdominal pain so severe that you don't want to move or temperatures that spike suddenly are signs of something more serious going on.

Even if your symptoms seem on the minor rather than the major end of the scale, if you are feeling anxious about the emerging signs and symptoms, it is probably a good time to call.

Below are some of the symptoms of IBD that could prompt a call to the doctor:

Severe symptoms
○ Diffuse yet intense abdominal pain that makes moving difficult
○ Wavelike abdominal pain associated with eating that may be diffuse to begin with but will localize, can be accompanied by nausea and vomiting, and may cause agitation
○ Great loss of blood in a short period of time that can be accompanied by dizziness or fainting
○ Sudden fever above 102 degrees F that can be accompanied by chills
○ Protracted nausea and vomiting
○ Profuse diarrhea that leads to symptoms of dehydration

Mild to moderate symptoms
○ Increase in diarrhea
○ Rectal pain that makes sitting uncomfortable
○ Slight increase in bleeding
○ Increase in cramping
○ Fever less than 102 degrees F
○ An emerging tender spot on the abdomen
○ Any symptoms related to ailments that accompany IBD, as listed in the Learning portion of this chapter

Before calling the doctor

Procedures, vacations, and weekends can all get in the way of reaching that trusted physician in a time of need. If your doctor is in a multi-physician practice, you may be able to reach his or her associate but not him or her directly. Whoever you reach may not be aware of your case or unable to recall specific details at 2 A.M., so it is important to anticipate the questions the doctor will likely ask and be prepared to answer them before calling.

Before making the call, write down all of the names of the medications you are taking, the amount you are taking of each one, and how often you are taking them. Be honest. If you aren't regularly taking your medication, now is the time to tell. Don't let the doctor think that you are taking your sixteen Pentasa tablets, four pills four times a day, if you haven't cracked the bottle in the past week or more. Also, record the name and telephone number of your regular pharmacy; at night or on holidays, have the telephone number of a pharmacy that is open during those times.

Then, briefly describe in writing the kinds of symptoms you are having. Don't say, "I am bleeding a lot." Instead, describe in amounts, "I lose a couple of teaspoons of blood each time I go" or "I think I lost about half a cup of blood." Don't say that you think you have a fever. Instead, take your temperature and write down the number that appears. It helps to jot down all of the symptoms, as it is easy to become flustered when speaking on the phone with the doctor.

Think back as to when the symptoms began and how you were feeling before they started. In the case of an elevated temperature, quickly think about other family members who may have been sick in the past week or so. This last bit of information will be helpful in attempting to get to the root of the problem, be it bacterial, viral, or disease activity.

You may want to quickly weigh yourself as well since the dosage of any additional medication prescribed over the phone will depend on how much you weigh. This is not a time for exaggeration. Be honest about your weight and try not make your symptoms sound greater or less than they really are. Being objective at a time like this may be difficult, but is vitally important.

Try to remember all you have eaten in the past forty-eight hours. That bowl of bran you swallowed in the morning or the extra rare hamburger you devoured two nights ago may also have more to do with your symptoms than the disease itself.

Making the call

Be sure to always have the phone number of your doctor either with you or memorized. The doctor, a receptionist, or a medical assistant will likely ask you for all of the information you have recorded prior to the call.

The doctor will decide whether the symptoms warrant immediate care or whether an office visit can be scheduled within the day or week. Often-times, he or she may try to see you in the office within the day or may pre-scribe new medication over the phone.

In the case of severe symptoms, you may be tempted to skip the call and head right to the closest emergency room. That is completely understand-able and is a judgment only you can make. However, you may still want to take the time to talk to your doctor first before heading to the hospital so he or she can call ahead to the ER doctors, alert them of your impending arrival, and give orders for your care.

Whether you are heading to the doctor's office or being whisked away to the emergency room, be sure to take all of the information you recorded prior to the phone call. You may have to repeat it to a few individuals before you are finally treated.

A few more words on calling the doctor: If you feel anxious about mak-ing a call to the doctor because you fear how he or she will react, it may be time to get a new doctor. A doctor should respond with concern or comfort, not with anger or hostility.

IN A SENTENCE:

> Call your doctor when your symptoms dictate, but be prepared with
> the relevant information prior to calling.

learning

The Ailments
That Accompany IBD

AS IF having the disease and being exposed to the various intestinal complications isn't enough, one in every four individuals with IBD will at some time or another have a systemic or extraintestinal manifestation of the disease that involves some other part of the body outside of the gastrointestinal tract. Commonly found in the skin, the bones, the joints, the blood, the liver and biliary system, the kidneys, and the eyes, these related conditions range from benign to life-threatening.

Some conditions affect largely those with CD or largely those with UC but some conditions strike all with IBD equally. Some of the conditions happen only when disease activity is high and subside with remission or removal of their colon or diseased intestinal segment. Still more conditions act as a harbinger of disease activity to come. Of course, some individuals report extraintestinal occurrences when they have no bowel disease activity at all. It is important to know that all of these systemic manifestations are reported in individuals who have never been diagnosed with bowel disease at all but may have some other illness.

What is known about these illnesses is that they are much more commonly reported in people with IBD than in the general public. However, what is not known is *why* these illnesses happen in greater numbers in people with IBD. It is suspected that in some cases, rogue GI immune cells circulate in the blood stream and attack far off tissues, bones, joints, and organs, causing a similar inflammatory response in the affected areas. Another theory suggests that a dysfunctional immune system indiscriminately attacks various areas. Still another theorizes that these, too, are genetic manifestations.

Because these side illnesses are so diverse and the list of them so expansive, an entire book could be dedicated to their various potential causes and treatments. For the purposes of this book, we will focus on the major areas that are affected and the different manifestations seen there. We will start from what can be seen and felt on areas visible to the eye and move inward to the blood, the bones, and the internal organs of the liver, the gallbladder, the pancreas, and the kidneys.

The skin

A relatively common site for manifestations of a slew of different diseases and bacterial and viral infections, the skin is also a frequent location for the various side ailments that affect individuals with IBD.

One of the most common manifestations in the skin is **erythema nodosum.** These red- to reddish-purple bumps most often appear on the lower legs such as the shins but can appear anywhere on the arms and legs and reportedly have also arisen in out-of-the-way areas such as the breasts. To the touch, they can be hot and hard, like a raised bruise, and can be as small as a pencil eraser or as large as the circumference of a soda can. Occurring more often in women than in men and slightly more commonly in CD than UC (although some would say the opposite is true), these unfortunate sore spots can last up to six weeks, either during or presaging disease activity. Unfortunately, there is no treatment but the passage of time to make these painful but benign bumps go away faster.

Erythema nodosum happens in IBD and other suspected autoimmune diseases like sarcoidosis, with a variety of viral illnesses including mononucleosis, streptococcus, hepatitis B, and tuberculosis, or as a reaction to medications like sulfa drugs or antibiotics like penicillin. Although there is usually nothing a doctor can do about these, it is important to report the appearance of the bumps.

A skin condition with the potential for serious danger is the appearance of **pyoderma gangrenosum.** Meaning literally pus in the skin, pyoderma lesions appear in less than 10 percent of UC patients. In CD patients, it appears to a much lesser degree and usually in individuals with at least some colonic involvement. Usually, this disease activity starts on the tops of the feet or lower legs but can appear anywhere on the body, in any size from one to 30 centimeters in diameter. They start with a sore area that develops a pimple-like formation that can fill with pus and blood. The sores rarely disappear on their own and often spread, eroding the skin in the area so that it can appear as a large, oozing, red wound. It is very important to report these to your doctor as soon as they appear.

Pyoderma gangrenosum appears in other immune-compromised individuals such as the elderly; however, studies have found that about half of its victims have underlying bowel disease. Mostly, the treatment for those with bowel disease is to avoid infection of the sore-like areas and to treat the underlying inflammation. Skin grafts can be performed to replace the damaged skin in some individuals.

Another common skin condition is the occurrence of enterocutaneous (intestines to skin) fistulas. These pesky channels mentioned in Day 5 can range from mildly annoying to very serious. Affecting mainly CD patients, the fistulas most commonly burrow from the rectum or anus through to the vagina, the buttocks, or the skin in and around that area. These abnormal tunnellike formations often leak pus or fecal matter, a manageable inconvenience at the very least. However, occasionally the fistulas will form between the intestines and the skin in the abdominal area, making potentially dangerous pathways for bacteria not normally found in the intestines. In this instance, immediate medical or surgical intervention is usually called for.

Skin tags and anal fissures are fairly common occurrences in CD patients. The skin tags form when hemorrhoid swellings in and around the anus flare up, stretching the surrounding skin. When the painful swellings shrink, the flaplike skin around them thickens and remains in the anal and perianal area. These tags don't hurt but can act as a haven for wayward fecal matter that can irritate the skin. As annoying as they may be, many doctors suggest against removing them surgically. Anal fissures are tears in the skin in and around the anus that can crack and bleed. They feel sore when open and itchy as they heal. Using creams such as bacitracin can help ease the pain and heal the area, and doctors can prescribe other medications in stubborn cases.

In the mouth, oral lesions are usually related to CD activity and can appear as canker sore–like formations in the cheeks or more pronounced ulcerations. There are tetracycline medications that can be swished in the mouth, but over the counter treatments such as painkilling topical preparations for toothaches and gum pain or simply dabbing the sore with hydrogen peroxide and milk of magnesia can help to soothe and heal the sores. The sores should be brought to the doctor's attention.

Sometimes, skin conditions are caused by the medications used to treat IBD or the nutritional status of the individual. Ugly but painless stretch marks from prednisone or the more worrisome oral erosion from 6-MP or azathioprine (Imuran, Azasan) are just two examples of this. As for nutrition, ulcerations on the lips, the swelling of the tongue or the appearances of red scaly patches on the skin are skin conditions that occur in individuals who are malnourished due to IBD activity.

The eyes

Often called the portals to the soul, the eyes also provide the doctor and the patient with a great view, so to speak, of an extraintestinal manifestation of IBD in both UC and CD patients. The following conditions are generally more rare than the skin manifestations and usually accompany both arthritic conditions such as **ankylosing spondilitis** and skin conditions like erythema nodosum.

Iritis and **uveitis** are technically two separate conditions, but they share the same symptoms and the same potential for loss of a degree of vision in the eye. Iritis is the inflammation of the iris, a translucent, circular disc that is punctuated by the pupil; the pigment under the iris determines if we have baby blues, soft browns, or anything in between. In iritis, patients have headaches, feel eye pain that ranges from very achy to somewhat sharp, experience an increased sensitivity to light, tear more often, and see slightly less sharp images. Uveitis is the inflammation of the uvea, a slightly larger, fibrous area that includes the iris as well as some surrounding structures and layers. In this condition, the area in front of the lens fills with pus, the pupil is abnormally opened, and there is inflammation around the cornea.

The danger of these conditions is that scar tissue can form from the inflammation and can cause vision loss called glaucoma. To diagnose these conditions, an ophthalmologist uses a special microscope to see into the eyes as the patient rests their chin in a bracing device. To treat the condition, eye drops containing steroids are administered for about ten days to reduce the inflammation. Eye pain can be eased with acetaminophen, warm and wet washcloths placed gently on the affected eye, or by using a patch to keep the eye closed.

Episcleritis is another, more benign condition of the eye related to IBD. The scleris is the white of the eye and episcleritis is an inflammation of this area. The pain associated with this is more burning and itchy in nature, causing tearing. More common in CD, episcleritis can be more frightening to others who may assume that what you have is a nasty case of conjunctivitis and want to steer clear of everything you touch. The treatment is the same as above.

The bones and joints

One of the most common subsets of conditions related to IBD involves rheumatologic disease, including the bones, the joints, and the connective tissues and spaces. Up to one-fourth of all IBD patients experience these aches and pains at least once and commonly on a regular basis, with or without signs of active disease.

Peripheral arthritis is perhaps the most common, happening equally in CD and UC to about one in five IBD patients. It appears mostly in the large joints of the extremities such as the knees and ankles in the legs, and the elbows, wrists, and shoulders in the arms. The joints tend to be painful, swell to varying degrees, are warm to the touch, and stiff to move. The symptoms can last a day or more than a year but the vast majority resolve in under eight weeks. In some patients with UC, the condition clears up with the removal of the diseased colon but it is never a primary consideration for a colectomy.

Peripheral arthritis is different from rheumatoid arthritis, a painful autoimmune disorder in which immune cells inflame joint linings and results in bone and joint deformities. Interestingly, however, some of the same medications used to treat IBD—steroids, methotrexate, Remicade, and Humira—are used to treat rheumatoid arthritis.

Usually, a doctor will examine the joint, perhaps taking X-rays to rule out any possible breaks due to bones weakened by malabsorption of calcium. In cases where IBD is not present, many individuals find relief from ibuprofen, naproxen, and other nonsteroidal anti-inflammatory drugs (NSAIDs); conversely, acetaminophen is usually prescribed for those with IBD, as NSAIDs have been shown to cause relapses and the worsening of symptoms in IBD. In the few years since the introduction of Cox-2 inhibitors like Vioxx and Celebrex, a few studies have indicated both improvement in IBD and exacerbation of IBD in patients taking these medications; that said, one exhaustive literature review on the subject published in a respected journal suggested that these drugs be avoided in IBD patients, as should other NSAIDs. (Merck took Vioxx off the market in 2004 because of a possible correlation with heart attacks. Celebrex, made by Pfizer, is still available.) Arthritis formula creams and gels applied to the skin above the affected joint, warm compresses or heating pads, long soaks in the bathtub, and alternating heat and cold can also relieve the pain associated with this condition.

Ankylosing spondilitis occurs more in CD than UC, in men more than women and begins mostly in patients under the age of thirty. It is a form of arthritis that causes pain and stiffness in the spine from inflammation of the spinal joints. The sacroiliac joint, the area where the spine and the pelvis meets in the lower back and buttocks, is commonly involved as are other areas of the body where tendons providing support for the joint connect and can become inflamed; these areas include the heels, the shins, the thighs, the rib cage, and the shoulder blades. People with ankylosing spondilitis feel a diffuse, sporadic pain in the lower back and buttocks, particularly in the morning. The vertebras slowly begin to fuse together as tiny bony outgrowths from one vertebra latch onto the next. The condition can progressively cause the fusion of the spine, one vertebra at a time, over several years, potentially causing deformity.

There may be a genetic component to ankylosing spondilitis as the individuals who have it typically carry an antigen known as HLA-B27. Having that tissue type does not mean that the carrier will have the disease; however, 6 percent of the population has that tissue type and more than 90 percent of those who have the tissue type have ankylosing spondilitis.

The diagnosis for this condition is difficult since X-ray findings may not show the effects of the condition for several years after the symptoms begin. Sometimes, doctors check the erythrocyte sedimentation rate for inflammation but the results of the test would not determine whether the inflammation was in the colon or in the spine so it is not reliable in IBD. Again, NSAIDs appear to help those who do not have IBD but may cause intestinal flareups in those with IBD; sulfasalazine, a drug used to treat IBD, has also been shown to be effective in reducing inflammation and may be a better option than the NSAIDs. Regular exercise helps to keep the joints fluid. Alternating heat with cold on the affected area can reduce some of the pain symptoms as can a dose of acetaminophen.

Sometimes the sacroiliac joint can become inflamed in IBD patients without the presence of ankylosing spondilitis. In this case, the antigen has little relevance, as this condition does not progressively affect the spine. The symptoms of low back and buttock pain are the same and are treated with acetaminophen as well as heat and cold therapy.

IBD and Your Bone Strength

I have a lot in common with my neighbor. We both love gardening, are both avid readers, both love animals, and are both active in our community. And we both also have low bone mass. While she fits the typical profile of a person with low bone mass (over fifty-five, female, Caucasian), I share the second and third feature but am only thirty-eight.

But I have IBD, now a known factor for accelerated bone loss in both men and women. In fact, it is estimated that between 30 and 60 percent of UC and CD patients have lower bone density than the rest of the population. Conditions such as osteoporosis (bone porosity), osteopenia (bone poverty), and osteomalacia (bone softness) not only happen in higher percentages among those with IBD, they happen several decades earlier than they do in the general population, starting in one's twenties and thirties as opposed to one's fifties and sixties.

Our skeletons are constantly forming, though at different rates during our lives. Two essential processes alternate—bone resorption and bone formation—to create strong bones with greater density. Resorption involves the dissolving of the bones, while formation follows closely, building the bones back up. These processes also allow us to store calcium in our bones and maintain healthy levels of calcium in the blood. But as we age, the processes slow down and the bones begin to lose calcium faster than it can be replaced, leading to more porous bones and to a greater potential for bone fractures.

One major and obvious reason for this is that people with both CD and UC are usually prescribed steroids at some point in their treatment, if not for years. The steroids interfere with the bone building process in the body by reducing the amount of calcium that is absorbed, increasing the amount of calcium that leaves the body through diarrhea, decreasing the amount of bone protective hormone estrogen, and altering the amount of bone resorption and bone formation in a negative balance. Any of these factors alone would reduce bone density in a healthy individual, but all of them combined cause a relatively rapid loss of density.

In certain cases, steroid use can lead to the death of bone, a condition called avascular necrosis. This extremely painful condition usually occurs in the hips or knees; because dead bone cannot be regenerated, the only treatment for this condition is joint replacement surgery.

Crohn's patients in particular are at risk for greater bone density loss, whether steroids were used to control the disease or not. In fact, a recent study found that those who were "steroid-naïve," meaning those who had never had steroids, had levels of low bone density similar to those who had used the drugs. One major reason for this is cytokine activity related to inflammation. Cytokines are a part of the inflammatory cycle in CD patients and also act to disrupt the resorption and formation activities in the bones. Also at fault are malabsorption problems associated with disease in the small intestines. Inflammation or loss of small intestine to surgery here can hamper the absorption of calcium and vitamin D, essential mineral and vitamin elements in the bone-building process.

To diagnose osteoporosis, osteopenia, and osteomalacia, a Dual Energy X-ray Absorptiometry (DEXA) scan can be performed (see Month 5). To prevent these conditions, your doctor may prescribe adequate amounts of calcium with vitamin D, either in the diet or in supplements, as well as biphosponate medications (see Week 3).

The liver and the biliary system

The liver and the supporting biliary system have been said to be the refinery in the body. The liver takes the components of food, medicines, and other chemicals we ingest or absorb through our lungs or skin and breaks them down, sending the materials to areas where they are needed in blood cells that are stored there. It also filters out the potentially harmful elements in the body, sending them out in the waste. The liver produces bile salts, acids, and cholesterol that are stored in the gallbladder until they are needed to help to break down digested fat; the salts are later reabsorbed in the ileum to be returned to the liver and used again. The pancreas is attached to the same common bile duct as the liver and the gallbladder and also delivers enzymes into the intestines to break down food.

There are so many other functions of the liver, about five hundred in all, that it is impossible to list them all here. So great is the liver's diversity in function that a man-made assistance device (think ventricle assist devices or kidney dialysis) has not been created to sustain an individual for more than a brief period of time. While the gallbladder can be removed (allowing contents it formerly stored to trickle into the duodenum), the pancreas, like the liver, must remain to manufacture enzymes. Because this system is so essential to life, the ramifications of IBD-related conditions in those organs could be mild to devastating, depending on the condition.

Perhaps the most benign but also the most common liver condition is fatty liver disease (**hepatic steatosis**), occurring with equal frequency in UC and CD patients. Both drug interactions from steroid therapy and malnutrition have been suggested as causes, but no one knows for sure why it happens. It tends to be directly related to the severity of the illness and can disappear as the disease goes into remission. That is why there is no treatment for it or any need to aggressively diagnose it, though it may show up in a liver biopsy or on an X-ray as an enlarged liver.

A more devastating, but thankfully less common, biliary complication known as **primary sclerosing cholangitis** (PSC) occurs in greater number in individuals who have UC than in CD; when it does occur in CD, it happens rarely in cases with colonic involvement of the disease. More men than women with IBD have the disease and IBD patients as a whole make up about half of all PSC patients. This disease occurs when the bile ducts both in and out of the liver become inflamed, causing scar tissue to form. As this occurs, the scar tissue blocks the pathway for bile and waste that then backs up in the liver, causing jaundice, weight loss, nausea, and itching as the predominant symptoms. A progressive disease, it can lead to the buildup of scar tissue within the liver, which impairs its function and is only rectified surgically with a liver transplant. Occasionally, as was the case with the late, great Chicago Bears running back Walter Payton, the condition may lead to the development of liver cancer or cancer of the bile ducts. When cancer is present, transplantation is not an option.

PSC is diagnosed with the use of an endoscopic procedure known as endoscopic retrograde cholangiopancreatography (ERCP). In this procedure, the endoscopic device is threaded through the mouth, down the esophagus, through the stomach, and into the intestines to the site where the common bile duct meets with the duodenum. There, the doctor should be able to see into the duct and find the scar tissue and resulting strictures in the bile duct. Also, certain blood markers may flag the presence of the disease. Unfortunately, there is no medical cure for this condition; however, some people find success in slowing its progression through the ingestion of a bile salt known as urso, or ursodeoxycholic acid.

Because the ileum is frequently the site of CD activity, the uptake of bile salts may be impaired. When this occurs, the liver can create more. At times, it is not enough and the levels of bile salts, bile acids, and cholesterol within the gallbladder are off kilter. The cholesterol begins to crystallize, slowly forming a stone; the process is called cholelithiasis. The smaller stones then get stuck in the mouth of the gallbladder, a four-inch long, eggplant-shaped sack attached below the liver to the common bile duct. The obstruction of the gallbladder causes intense pain that is associated with eating, particularly in the case of fatty meals. People with gallbladder pain usually describe it as being a stabbing pain in the middle of their chest traveling to the back or the shoulder, often accompanied by nausea and vomiting. At times, these stones can cause an infection to form, leading to fever as a symptom. In some individuals, the stones cause no problems but in others it is suspected that these asymptomatic stones can lead to gallbladder cancer.

Ultrasound can show the presence of the stones while certain enzymes on blood tests will appear to be elevated. Other diagnostic tests involving the use of imaging devices and injected contrast solutions are helpful. Usually, removal of the gallbladder is recommended, as the condition is irreversible.

Pancreatitis may also be related to gallstones or can occur as a medication side effect with immunosuppressive therapy. With gallstones, a stone travels down the common bile duct past the area where the pancreas joins. The stone then becomes lodged in the duct, allowing none of the enzymes to pass. Nausea, vomiting, fever, and strong abdominal pain usually follow.

Although this condition is rare, it is potentially very serious. In the case of gallstones, it is treated using the ERCP. In that procedure, the physician uses the endoscopic instrument to make a small slit in the opening of the bile duct to allow the passage of the stone, which is then collected in a tiny basket and withdrawn from the patient. In the case of medication-induced pancreatitis, the medication may be discontinued, with the doctor prescribing a different course of medical therapy instead.

The kidneys

Like the liver, the kidneys act as filters for the blood, sifting out about two quarts of water and other waste by-products each day. These two organs, located just below the rib cage in the center of the back, shuttle the waste out of the body through the ureters, little connections between the organs and the bladder. From there, the body dispenses the waste as urine. Unlike the liver, kidneys can be helped to function by means of a man-made system called dialysis when disease activity diminishes the kidneys' capacity. Thankfully, the amount of IBD complications related to the kidney are relatively small, being confined to small percentages of CD patients.

Amyloidosis is a potentially serious condition related to IBD that can cause irreversible damage to the kidneys. It affects about one percent of CD patients and far fewer UC patients, appearing irrespective of disease activity. This condition happens in several areas of the body when waxy proteins called amyloid are deposited in organ tissues. Where the danger usually results is when these proteins make their way to the kidneys and disrupt function, leading to kidney failure.

One sign of the disease is an elevated amount of protein in the urine, called proteinuria. From that finding, a biopsy can then be taken of the kidney to confirm the diagnosis. Some success in slowing or halting the disease has been found in the drug combination of prednisone and melphalan while others have used colchicines. As the disease progresses, dialysis with later kidney transplantation may be necessary.

Kidney stones, the formation of which is known as nephroliathiasis, occur in CD patients, primarily those with extensive ileal disease or ileal resection. There are a few reasons as to why these happen. The first is that the digestive process in the diseased ileum is disrupted enough for fatty acids to join with calcium and be excreted in the fecal matter, leaving high amounts of fat to be found in the fecal matter. The problem arises when oxalate, which usually couples with calcium, is left unpartnered and finds its way to the kidneys in excessive amounts that cause the stones to form. Another reason is that the balance of acid in the urine is disrupted, causing an imbalance that a different kind of stone to form.

When conditions appear ripe for such a situation to occur, it usually results in intense pain. Like the gallstones, these stones tend to get stuck in the passageways, producing a sharp, cramping pain that radiates down the back. Nausea and vomiting are common as well and sometimes the person with the stone will see blood in their urine. The stones can be located on an X-ray or with a sonogram and usually resolve themselves, passing into the urine stream. Extracorporeal shockwave lithotripsy, a procedure in which small shock waves are sent through a tub of water in which the patient is sitting, may also help to break up bigger stones so they can be passed. Drinking lots of water helps to pass the stones and adopting a low fat, low oxalate diet can reduce the chance of recurrence.

Hydronephrosis happens when the ureters are blocked, not allowing the usual flow of waste to travel to the bladder. The waste then remains and builds up in the kidneys. If it is not resolved, scar tissue forms in the kidneys, causing kidney failure in some cases. In IBD, this happens most frequently in CD when ileal disease puts pressure on the ureter. The symptoms of this are a dull pain in the area of the kidneys as well as the presence of blood or pus in the urine.

A diagnosis of the condition utilizes X-rays and an injected contrast solution. To treat the condition, the ureters may have to be dilated and the diseased segment of ileum removed to reduce further pressure.

Another IBD-related situation within the urinary tract is related to an intestinal complication, the formation of a fistula from the intestine to a ureter or the bladder. As mentioned in Day 5, these occur in CD patients, more commonly in men than women. Symptoms of the condition include fecal matter exiting in the urine, air passing through the urinary opening, and blood appearing in the urine. To treat the condition, resection surgery to remove the fistulous tract and the diseased intestinal segment is required if medical treatment fails to close the fistula.

The blood

Our blood is a rich source of information about anything that is going on in our bodies, right or wrong. With IBD, this is no different. Our doctors can tell with erythrocyte sedimentation rates if inflammation is causing a problem in our guts. They can see if our liver levels are normal or if there is something amiss bacterially with an elevated white count.

But IBD patients' blood can also be affected by a condition known as **hypercoagulation**, meaning blood clots can more easily form. Clots can affect UC and CD patients equally and are found most often in the legs, more often than not in bedridden patients. The clots present as tender areas that can be hot and hard to the touch.

Doctors can locate these clots using a contrast solution that is injected into the veins where the suspected clot resides. X rays are then taken and can show where the blockage exists. Filters can be placed in the veins and anticoagulant medication such as heparin can be administered.

One note: Don't think a blood clot can't happen to you. On Memorial Day 2005, I awoke with strong waves of abdominal pain. After a few of the usual GI tests turned up no reason for the pain and the pain intensified, I was sent to surgery. There, my surgeon discovered that a Crohn's-free loop of ileum had been strangled of its blood supply by an errant clot. The dead loop was resected. I had not been bedridden, nor was the clot in the most common place, nor did I have a family history of clotting conditions. Instead, my physicians feel the clot was related to Crohn's. Because I now have a known tendency for hypercoagulation, I can no longer take certain medications, such as hormone-based birth control or most migraine medication.

Anemia is often a symptom of CD and UC, caused most commonly by intestinal bleeding. Also, the condition may be caused by poor absorption of vitamin B_{12} in CD patients with severe ileal disease or extensive ileal resection. Some symptoms of anemia include fatigue, pale skin, an increased sensitivity to temperature changes, confusion, and dizziness; one odd symptom is the curvature of fingernails. A blood test measuring hemoglobin and albumin can reveal low levels, a classic sign of anemia. To treat the condition, a diet rich in foods containing iron or iron supplements are prescribed, as may be vitamin B_{12} shots or nasal spray.

Sometimes, blood levels can be altered by the medications taken for the treatment. While white cell suppression is the goal of immunosuppressive therapy, certain liver enzymes may be missing or not produced enough to break down the toxic parts of the medication, leading to dangerously low levels of white cells, red cells, and/or platelets. The body then becomes acutely susceptible to infections that it is no longer able to battle. Once the immunosuppressive therapy is withdrawn or reduced, the blood levels should return to near normal. Certain blood-cell-promoting medications, such as Neupogin for white cell promotion or Epogen for red cell promotion, can sometimes be prescribed to boost blood levels.

Other possible complications

As a whole, doctors sporadically report what are called case studies. Individuals whose symptoms, disease activity, or treatment responses are unusual will have their medical information written into a report that then appears in medical journals for the purpose of sharing what might be a once in a lifetime occurrence with others. In the case of extraintestinal manifestations of IBD, this is no different. These case studies serve to highlight the rare cases of rare systemic manifestations of relatively rare diseases. Such case studies have reported on suspected links to IBD with such cardiac illness as giant cell myocarditis, lung occurrences like bronchiolitis and interstitial lung disease, and other random symptoms such as seemingly related inflammation of the vulva. It is important to share information in this way in case other physicians who have had scattered experiences see these reports and possibly are able to record yet another manifestation. It is also essential to remember that these are rare conditions and about as likely to happen to you as getting struck by lightning.

IN A SENTENCE:

Both CD and UC patients may experience many, varied symptoms of the disease in different areas of the body.

Coping with Pain

AS YOU have probably figured out by now, pain is inherent in IBD. Muscle pain, back pain, rectal pain, oral pain, abdominal pain, sharp pain, cramping pain, wave-like pain, pain that keeps you up at night, pain that prevents you from eating, pain from surgery, pain from shots or intravenous lines, pain from headaches caused by medication, pain from the extraintestinal manifestations like joint pain or painful skin nodules. And this doesn't even address the emotional and financial pain you may encounter with IBD.

While it may seem at times that the only thing that doesn't hurt is your hair, I promise you that this pain will come and go. There are medications to take and things to do to make the pain go away or at least make it tolerable.

Pain medications

The first line of defense in management of joint pain, fever, and muscle aches are over the counter treatments you can purchase in just about any drug store. The name brands of these medications should be as familiar to you as the names of your own relatives: Tylenol, Bayer, Advil, and Aleve. But are they all the same? And if they aren't, do any of these have potential side effects that might complicate IBD? The answers are no and yes, in that order.

Tylenol's chief ingredient is acetaminophen, a fever- and pain-reducing medication used for the relief of minor aches and pains, headaches, and muscle aches. It can be taken in four doses of one gram each (usually two 500 mg pills), four to six hours apart, not exceeding four grams in twenty-four hours; some formulas last for eight hours, so it is important to read the label for dosing instructions. It should not be taken with alcohol as it can cause liver damage. In those with preexisting liver disease or liver damage, it should be taken in lower doses prescribed by a doctor since it has been known to lead to liver failure and death in those with these preexisting conditions. Additionally, acetaminophen is contained in numerous multi-symptom allergy, cold, and flu remedies, so use caution to avoid overdosing when mixing different medications containing acetaminophen.

For those with IBD, acetaminophen is blessedly gentle on the GI tract and effective in lowering fever associated with inflammation or abscess, reducing joint pain, and soothing muscle aches and pain from random sites such as oral lesions and erythema nodosum. Some individuals, however, do not find the relief they need for easing strong joint pains.

The next three medications, aspirin (Bayer and other brands), ibuprofen (Advil, Motrin IB, and other brands) and naproxen (Aleve and other brands), fall in the category of non-steroidal anti-inflammatory drugs (NSAIDs), medications that help to lower fever and ease muscle aches and inflammation. These drugs have been especially beneficial for individuals who suffer from joint pain and inflammation associated with arthritis, but they have been found to cause gastrointestinal bleeding in some individuals. These medications are also common ingredients in multisymptom allergy, cold, and flu remedies, so it is worth reading the label for the active ingredients to avoid overdose.

In people with IBD, some patients with active disease taking the medications for joint pain experienced a worsening of their symptoms, while others who were in clinical remission had a relapse. Other individuals experience neither worsening of their symptoms nor relapse. For these reasons, it is important for individuals with CD or UC to consult with their doctor first before taking the medication.

Certain IBD symptoms may be aided with the application of topical over the counter medications. Individuals with arthritis—those with and without IBD—find some relief in using creams rubbed on affected joints; the creams (Tiger Balm, Ben-Gay, Icy Hot) usually contain menthol and an aspirin-like medication and work by generating the feeling of heat at the site by increasing blood flow to the area. For anal and rectal pain, hemorrhoid creams (Preparation H, Anusol HC) help to shrink swollen, painful tissues.

Many pain medications called narcotics require a prescription from a physician. Codeine, Demerol, morphine, Vicodin, Dilaudid, and a number of other medications are used in pill, injection, and inhalable forms for the relief of severe pain associated with abscesses, surgeries, obstructions, and major joint pain in individuals with IBD. All of these drugs carry risk of addiction, overdose, and dangerous interaction with some medications and alcohol; the use of narcotic pain relievers should be discussed at length with a physician prior to taking the medication. Also, some formulas of these drugs contain either acetaminophen or ibuprofen and patients using these medications should be careful to avoid an accidental overdose of acetaminophen and ibuprofen.

One benefit of using some narcotic medications is that they tend to slow the bowels, thus reducing the incidence of diarrhea. While this may seem like a boon for some, it may actually act to mask progression of the disease by limiting pain sensation and bowel activity. If you have to use such medications, be sure to talk to the doctor about how long you can expect to be on them.

Relief beyond pills

Not all relief can be found in the shape of a pill. Centuries before pharmaceutical companies mixed their magic formulas, the health gurus of many communities used other methods to control pain and inflammation, all with varying degrees of success.

The use of heat and cold is one of the most common ways of reducing pain and inflammation, especially in the joints. Heat promotes circulation and relaxation and can ease movement in a stricken joint. Moist heat— through the use of a warm and moist compress or a dip in a warm bath or hot tub—is particularly helpful in easing the pain and tension caused by an abscess or aching muscles. Cold packs can reduce inflammation and pain in tender joints. Alternating the two treatments in regular intervals can reduce inflammation and pain in many individuals, experts find.

There is some caution people should take in administering such treatment. First, make sure that the heat or cold is not administered directly to the skin; instead, make sure the element (a cold pack, a heating pad) is covered with a soft cloth to prevent damage to the skin. Using heat or cold on skin damaged by a burn, a cut, or at an injection site may also cause further damage. Second, give the area a rest. Sustained heat or cold therapy can cause tissue injury. Some experts find that placing cold and then heat in that sequence three times in a row will reduce inflammation and pain if done two to three times in a day.

Thinking the pain away through meditation or imagery has been documented to help individuals with pain related to cancer and its treatments. One particularly relaxing form of meditation involves closing the eyes, clearing the mind of any distractions, progressively allowing muscles to go slack, and focusing on breathing deeply for several minutes. Imagery incorporates the relaxation techniques of meditation, yet allows the practitioner to travel in their minds to an image of a desirable, safe, comfortable place. Both of these techniques have been shown to slow heart rate, relax muscles, decrease pain perception, improve circulation, and release tension in a variety of studies.

Rubbing the pain away through massage is also a well-documented pain management technique that improves circulation, relaxes muscles, releases tension, and decreases pain perception. There are a number of massage techniques and nearly all of them involve one individual touching another. Aside from communicating love and caring, touch has been shown to be physically beneficial for individuals suffering from cancer and other illnesses.

Moving the pain away through gentle exercise such as tai chi or yoga can aid in pain relief. When IBD strikes, the tendency is to remain within close proximity of a bathroom, curled in a fetal position. But most patients find that such gentle exercise can be done safely during flare-ups—often within reach of the toilet. Studies have shown that people who exercise even in modest amounts share the benefits of reduced tension, reduced stress, increased circulation, and increased energy, all things on which pain has the opposite effect. Most individuals can participate in light exercise, but you should consult with your doctor before taking up any increased physical activity. Also, concentrating on performing the correct moves can help to take your mind off the pain.

Other Eastern-based practices, acupuncture and acupressure, have found greater acceptance in pain relief, particularly in postoperative pain. The methods are based on ancient Chinese beliefs that energy patterns within the body exist and are the source of pain when they are disrupted. Through the insertion of long, slender, metal needles into certain points of the body, it is believed by the practitioners of acupuncture that the energy flow can be restored and thus pain is relieved. Acupressure involves a similar theory but instead of using needles, the practitioner presses certain reflexive spots on the body called meridians. The feeling is that by deeply pressing these points, certain chemicals are released in the brain and cause a reduction in pain. Both of these methods are controversial and difficult to study, but in some major medical institutions they are considered to be credible forms of therapy and are offered to patients in addition to medical treatment.

Biofeedback is a relatively new invention in the scheme of medical history. This therapy involves placing electrodes on certain areas of the body to record involuntary activity such as involuntary muscular contractions, internal body temperature, heart rate, and blood pressure. Through several sessions, the individual is taught to anticipate these changes and make corrections through a degree of mind control over the affected body part. Though this approach is controversial, some individuals with irritable bowel syndrome as well as IBD have found relief using this technique.

IN A SENTENCE:

> *Pain relief can come in a bottle but also through the use of alternative methods.*

learning

Genetics and Other Causative Factors of IBD

AT THE moment you are reading this, no one knows for certain what causes CD or UC. Researchers don't think anyone will know for sure for a decade or longer.

That said, theories abound for the possible genetic and environmental causes of the diseases, together and individually. Researchers puzzle over why certain people with no genetic history get it, while some families establish clear patterns. They look at segments of society and wonder why the diseases primarily occur in modern, industrial societies, while those living in the bush escape unscathed. Could it be rogue genes that create impaired, dysfunctional immune systems? Could it be invasive bacteria? What about a combination of the two?

Because scientists are unable to explain the why of the diseases, it is difficult to come up with a way to stop or to cure them. Even with genetic markers, it is nearly impossible to develop blood tests that can predict who will be at a high risk of developing the disease and who is not. But just finding the cause of a disease does not necessarily mean that a cure will be found or a diagnostic test will be developed. However, knowing how the disease switches itself on may lead to a way to turn it off and keep it off. That is why it is crucial for the scientists to find the cause for the diseases.

The following are different theories scientists have studied in pursuit of the causation of IBD.

Food intolerances, allergies, and reactions

The idea that what we eat makes us who we are is a long held belief; in the world of IBD, that idea takes on particular meaning. After all, the food that is ingested, ground up, and absorbed or not absorbed passes over the very area where the disease occurs. What made food all the more suspicious is that the diet heavy in refined wheat and refined sugars of the Western world is not shared by those in the Eastern world, where more raw, whole foods are ingested and the IBD rate is rock bottom.

With that in mind, scientists did not make a huge leap in identifying food as a potential cause of IBD. Perhaps, some guessed, it is milk or its byproducts, wheat or its byproducts, or perhaps refined sugars that caused the gut's immune system to turn on itself. Margarine and eggs have also aroused suspicion. But proving these suspicions is another matter entirely, as the studies that suggest such links rarely involve more than two or three dozen individuals and are not replicated in other controlled instances. A large portion of these food probes are based on subjective impressions as well, leading other scientists to point out other subjectively gleaned inconsistencies to potentially debunk the theory. One such example of this is the theory of the Western diet versus the Eastern diet. In Japan and Israel, one could easily argue that the Eastern diet has greater influence, and yet the prevalence of CD and UC is moderately high and climbing.

Food allergies and intolerances are another story. Foods that cause the greatest amount of allergic reactions include shellfish, nuts, fish, wheat, milk, and eggs. However, clinically proven allergies occur in only three percent of children and one percent of adults, making the occurrence relatively rare. An actual allergic reaction involves the mast cells that are everywhere in the body but are common in the nose, the throat, the lungs, the skin, as well as the gastrointestinal tract. Because of this, the symptoms can include gastrointestinal events such as diarrhea, abdominal cramps, and vomiting, and also asthma and hives. The important item to remember about allergies is that the food and the reaction to it are related and that when the food is withdrawn, the reaction is not present. Studies that have suggested allergic reaction have not been able to prove the link.

One thing that should be mentioned here is the Specific Carbohydrate Diet, a formulation created by a scientist who was the mother of a UC patient. Working on the theory that certain carbohydrates contribute to certain substances that injure the intestine, the scientist created a diet that was devoid of these carbohydrates. Her daughter fared well on the diet and a book was written that exploded in popularity, especially among IBD patients who were desperate to find relief. On the Internet, there is no shortage of patient sites featuring testimonials from individuals who claim to be cured of not only IBD but also celiac sprue and autism as well.

That said, there has been no relevant research performed on the efficacy of the diet in IBD; a search of studies turned up only a case study involving two patients. Most of the IBD doctors with whom I have spoken point out several inconsistencies in the diet and the science on which it is based. Further, they say that the majority of their patients who have tried it found it too restrictive to remain on for any length of time, or derived little benefit from it. However, most of those doctors had no problems with their patients trying the diet as long as it was clear that it was discussed with them first and that medications would not be abandoned during that trial.

The MAP bacteria and/or other bacterial and viral infections

A long time ago, when researchers were first identifying CD, it was suggested that the disease was related to tuberculosis bacteria found in the intestines. Early reports suggest that as the tuberculosis in bovine herds dropped, the incidence rate of the tuberculosis of the intestines in humans dropped as well. Here we are more than half a century away from those reports and the suggestion of such an infection is again on the table for researchers to examine. The mycobacterium avium subspecies paratuberculosis, commonly shortened to mycobacterium paratuberculosis or MAP, is one of the chief suspects to be studied in recent years by animal and human medical experts alike.

The disease was found in animals that chew their cud and was caused by the bacteria in cows is known as Johne's (pronounced "Yo-nees") disease, the manifestation of which is strikingly similar to CD. Animals with the disease suffer from increasing degrees of weight loss, diarrhea, and malabsorption. Although the animals seemingly do not experience pain, they can become so thin that their bone structure shows through their hides. In animals that have died of the disease, samples of their intestines show the same granuloma formation as is present in patients with CD who have undergone resection surgery. The bacteria begins to multiply within the infected cow's intestines and is found in the fecal matter; later the bacteria works its way into the blood stream and is found in blood samples and in milk or colostrum.

Veterinary scientists believe the bacteria is passed from cow to cow through fecal matter that makes it into the food supply, something that is not hard to imagine as the cows' diarrhea can spread easily within animal living areas. The diarrhea can also make it to the teats, potentially infecting a nursing calf. There has also been some evidence of *in utero* transference of the bacteria as well. Approximately 22 percent of U.S. dairy herds and 8 percent of beef herds are infected with the bacteria.

The theory on human transference is that bacteria survive the pasteurization process and remain in milk consumed in humans. In fact, recently such bacteria were reportedly found in the United Kingdom in milk sold for human consumption. The theory continues by positing that the infected milk is consumed and the bacteria breach the epithelium where the immune system is unable to handle the intruder, causing pain, inflammation, and bleeding. Because the bacteria can live and reproduce in the intestines, it multiplies and spreads in different areas.

One Florida doctor has found that by treating CD patients with antimycobacterial drugs (rifabutin and macrolide) that the inflammation subsided and the wounded intestine healed. Another Australian physician is in the process of conducting a multicenter study on the effects of using antimicrobial medications (clarithromycin, rifabutin, and clofazimine) to treat an alleged MAP infection in Crohn's patients.

In the five years since the first edition of this book appeared, the controversy has deepened. Several scientists have reported newer, better ways of detecting the virus in the tissues of CD patients while others have postulated that there is a connection between the presence of the virus and the defect on chromosome 16, where the NOD2/CARD15 gene resides. Still, the naysayers maintain that there has yet to be large, credible, multicentered studies, the results of which can be repeated in different, independent locations. These voices of strong criticism point out that even with better detection methods, the studies have not been able to detect the virus in all of the Crohn's patients examined; in fact, the percentages are little more than half in most studies. Finally, these same scientists say that the antimycobacterial medications used in the therapy regimens used by some doctors would act on pathogens other than mycobacteria.

Whatever the case, many in the medical community are tiring over the seemingly ceaseless study and discussion over the MAP-Crohn's connection. As one highly respected researcher wrote in a recent paper on the subject, "If there is no evidence of a causal association of MAP and Crohn's disease, we need to direct resources to other avenues of research. This controversy has persisted far too long and needs to be expeditiously resolved."

As for other potential bacterial or viral causes of IBD, a number of suspects have emerged in the past forty years. It is a logical place to look for the cause, as such agents have been known to cause intestinal problems. *E. coli*, campylobacter, salmonella, and shigella are all bacteria that can cause serious, at times fatal, gastrointestinal symptoms. Paramyxovirus, Listeria monocytogenes, and Helicobacter hepaticus have been examined as possible pathogenic infections in CD and UC as well. A number of viruses have been examined as well. At one point, for example, cytomegalovirus was considered the chief suspect in UC, but then researchers thought that perhaps this opportunistic infection simply existed because the defense of the colon was weakened by the underlying disease. However, at this point, no evidence conclusively points to a bacterial or viral cause.

The MMR vaccine

The controversy of the link between the measles vaccine and the incidence of IBD heightened in the last decade as a small number of studies and reports were released on the topic internationally. One tiny study reported links between children exposed to the measles virus in utero and another reportedly found miniscule measles virus proteins in the bowel walls of CD patients.

Perhaps the most widely reported in this flurry of journal articles was the one that appeared in the British medical journal *Lancet* in 1998. In the article, the researchers connected the dots between the incidence of inflammatory bowel disease, behavioral disorders, and autism and the use of the vaccine, which also includes the vaccines for mumps and rubella (called the MMR vaccine, usually given in two separate doses between twelve and fifteen months and four and six years). The theory they put forth suggested that the vaccine caused inflammation in the digestive tract which led to increased intestinal permeability as well as decreased absorption of certain essential vitamins, minerals, and nutrients. This lack of nutrients led to the behavioral disorders and to the autism.

The uproar that followed the printing of this study was great, for already a suspected link had been made between autism and the use of vaccines. Detractors immediately denounced the study including one, whose editorial cited apprehension about the study that appeared in the same journal issue. At issue was that the patient population in the study was considered too small and not well selected (twelve patients total, all of whom were culled from a gastroenterology department in a hospital and therefore were known to have bowel disease), that there was no mention of finding the existence of the virus borne in the vaccine in the tissues of the brains or guts of the patients, and that the behavioral symptoms preceded the bowel symptoms. The study was not replicable, meaning that others could not duplicate the results and ties established within the original study. It also did not explain why the millions of children who received the vaccines did not have brain or bowel disorders.

In the United States, the Centers for Disease Control performed a population-based study in June 2000 and concluded that there was no link between the MMR vaccine and IBD. In the study, they looked at a number of factors, including the age at which the shot was given in both people with IBD and those without IBD. More than a handful of other studies have refuted the findings reported in the *Lancet* article while others were not able to duplicate the findings of the in utero measles exposure theory and the evidence of the measles virus in the bowel walls of CD patients.

The IL-23r, NOD2/CARD15, and other genetic affiliations

In recent years, scientists have been searching for a possible genetic link, understandably so as many individuals with either disease often have relatives with IBD. Twin studies, a common yardstick in the field of genetic studies, have shown that fraternal twins seem to have the same incidence rate of IBD as the rest of the immediate family but identical twins, those sharing the same genetic makeup, were found to have higher rates of occurrence. At the same time, no identical twins have ever been reported in medical literature where one has CD and the other has UC; this suggests that the diseases have similar but not identical genetic background.

Genetic registries of individuals who have CD or UC in their families have proven to be the basis of different studies involving the location of genes that may be related to IBD. One particularly exciting discovery took place in Pennsylvania in late October 2006. Researchers announced their finding that specific coding on a gene known as the interleukin-23 (IL-23) receptor located on chromosome 1p31 predisposed people to CD, and UC, while other variants in coding appeared to protect others from developing IBD. These same scientists believe that the differences in coding may also explain the occurrence of rheumatoid arthritis, the skin disease psoriasis, and multiple sclerosis, diseases not only linked with IBD through common treatments but also within families. The discovery, confirmed through multiple medical research facilities throughout the world, also provides direction for future medical advances, as it may point the way to targeted IL-23–based treatments.

In an earlier study, some of the same researchers in the United States and France used different methods to make a similar discovery in families where CD was documented to exist. They found that abnormalities existed on the NOD2/CARD15 gene, located on chromosome 16. The NOD2/CARD15 gene is found in a certain kind of cell called a monocyte, the job of which is to identify and destroy a relatively common bacteria.

So far, possible genetic links have been found on chromosomes 1, 3, 6, 7, 12, 14, 16, and 19. These researchers believe that this mutation may explain why the immune system seems to overreact, launching a prolonged attack that leads to the chronic inflammation and related symptoms.

The work on the genetic association of IBD continues.

Oral contraceptives

Could the sexual revolution of the mid-sixties have had an effect of the diagnosis rates of CD and UC? Enovid, the first oral contraceptive, and a harbinger of the so-called sexual revolution, debuted in 1960 and saw their peak usage in 1978, where the rate of use has remained fairly steady ever since. During the same time, more and more young women were being diagnosed with IBD. This possible link made curious researchers examine the possibility that the little pills might have an undesirable effect on the intestines.

In more than a handful of studies, researchers found an elevated incidence of IBD in those who took the Pill. However, one study did not find such a risk. But what wasn't explained was why men of the same age, children, and postmenopausal patients—presumably those not on the Pill—shared similar incident rates.

Parasites

Or should we say the lack thereof? When it was noticed that IBD appeared largely in Western cultures, scientists began to theorize exactly what part of Western culture might cause the disease. The Western diet was looked at for a long time, with no real culprit identified. Other environmental issues were examined, with nothing really emerging as the one true reason. Everyone seemed to look at what we had, instead of what we didn't have: worms.

Scientists at the University of Iowa Center for Digestive Diseases hit on a theory in the past decade that has sparked growing interest internationally. While Westerners had different clothes than those in the East, different food than those in the East, and different environmental conditions than those in the East, we no longer had intestinal worms with which children and adults in the East continued to wrestle. What was particularly interesting was that in nations that had low IBD rates in the past—Israel, Australia, and Japan to name a few—the rates rose when sanitation systems improved. Our modern water systems and up to date hygienic practices had all but eliminated the occurrence of intestinal worms. And when one slipped by and caused infection, medicine was developed to eradicate the parasites.

Perhaps, the researchers thought, that the worms actually enacted an immune response, known as the Th2 response. In individuals with IBD, the Th1 response is high but the Th2 response is low. In healthy individuals, the Th1 and Th2 response work together, sort of the yin and the yang of the immune response. To promote the Th2 response in IBD patients, a worm would have to be found that would not damage the intestines yet would still provoke the weakened immune response. When they did locate such a worm, a helminth, they fed the eggs to a small number of IBD patients. The response was encouraging in those with CD, with some of the patients able to wean themselves off all medication if they were given electrolyte solution laced with the eggs every three weeks.

The theory has yet to be proven conclusively. However, slightly larger studies have since been performed that found the best response in those with intact terminal ileums who were on immunosuppressives. Currently, the theory is being tested in a large, multicentered, placebo-controlled study.

Psychosomatics

Since the early days of UC and CD, opinions about the role of a mind-body connection in relation to IBD have played over and over. Prior to the 1960s, many physicians would send IBD patients to psychologists and psychiatrists, who in turn developed a psychological profile of the typical UC patient. A closer look at the studies that were published to support such theories showed serious flaws, including a lack of or appropriate control groups. As more and more medical evidence supported a more physiological illness of the intestines, the psychological theories lost ground.

Emotions certainly have an effect on the general health and well-being of everyone, IBD patients included. Stress and depression related to having and adjusting to a chronic illness can make symptoms worse, and a recent study in England showed that stress increased an inflammatory response in UC patients, leading researchers to theorize that stress plays a role in flareups. However, no conclusive link has been found to a psychological illness and the development of CD or UC.

Short chain fatty acids

In everyone, the presence of short chain fatty acids, formed when bacteria in the colon break down certain carbohydrates, is beneficial as these products help to maintain a strong epithelial barrier. These acids are formed when bacteria oxidate certain carbohydrates. However certain sulfides can reduce the production of such beneficial substances.

Due to this interaction, some scientists believe that the induction of these short chain fatty acids via enema can help to promote epithelial health. Additionally, some of these same scientists have found that the elimination from the diet of sulfur-producing foods such as eggs, milk, and cheese can reduce symptoms in those with UC.

Again, similar studies have not found these truths to be repeatable. Therefore, more study is needed in this area.

Smoking

Since 1982, the effect of smoking as a risk factor in the development of IBD has been studied with interesting results.

Researchers have found that a greater number of nonsmokers than smokers have UC. Among those who do smoke, disease flare-ups have been reported as the patient attempts to quit smoking; using a nicotine patch was found to be beneficial in reducing symptoms in a small study. Scientists theorize that there may be some protective natural ingredient in the tobacco that causes the UC to remain quiet.

But that doesn't begin to explain why the opposite is true in CD patients. Smoking has been found to cause flare-ups in patients with CD, and those who continue to smoke have greater disease activity than those who have never lit up.

Whatever the case, it is important for the patients not to start smoking, or to stop if they do smoke. The risks to the pulmonary and cardiovascular systems are not worth it.

IN A SENTENCE:

> *Both possible environmental and genetic causes of IBD have been and continue to be examined.*

FIRST-WEEK MILESTONE

By the end of your first week, you have begun to take control of your CD or UC as you have now:

○ LEARNED WHAT THE DISEASE IS AND WHAT IT IS NOT AS WELL AS HOW IT AFFECTS YOU THROUGH THE INTESTINES AND IN OTHER PARTS OF THE BODY.

○ VERIFIED YOUR DIAGNOSIS.

○ BEEN INTRODUCED TO THE POSSIBLE CAUSES OF THE DISEASE.

○ BECOME ACQUAINTED WITH THE GRIEVING PROCESS.

○ DISCOVERED THE IMPORTANCE OF AND HAVE THE WHEREWITHAL TO ASSEMBLE YOUR HEALTH CARE TEAM.

○ DEVELOPED COPING TECHNIQUES FOR THE PAIN.

The Role of Medication in the Treatment of IBD

BECAUSE THERE currently is no cure for IBD, the role of medication in the treatment of UC and CD is to control the symptoms of the inflammatory disease by altering the functions of certain cells in the body. Some of the medications have proved their value and safety through decades of use, while others have made smashing debuts in recent years.

The one thing that you should remember about these medications is that the only chance they have for having any effect on the disease is if they are taken exactly as prescribed. We'll talk in Week 3 about ways to remain compliant, but it is important to know right now that the drugs listed here will do you no good if you don't take them.

Sulfasalazine and related medications

If ever there were an old standby in the treatment of these diseases, it would have to be **sulfasalazine** (Azulfidine). A derivative of the sulfa drugs first created to treat infection on the battlefields of Europe, this drug marries the compounds of sulfapyridine and 5-aminosalicylic acid (5-ASA, also known as mesalamine or mesalazine). The reason for joining the two compounds is that 5-ASA, the therapeutic agent in IBD treatment, is absorbed quickly in the upper part of the intestines, never making it to the areas where it is designed to help. When ingested, the two ingredients remain intact until they enter the colon where bacteria break the bond that holds them together. From there, the sulfapyridine is absorbed, travels to the liver where it is broken down further, is delivered to the kidneys and is excreted in the urine. The 5-ASA heads into the epithelium where it changes slightly and begins to alter the cellular activities that take place in the inflamed area, leading to an overall decreased amount of inflammation. The 5-ASA is not greatly absorbed, tending to be more topical in its action; however, it must be noted that while the drug is relatively mild, some individuals require only the 5-ASA drugs for effective treatment of the disease.

A number of side effects can occur with sulfasalazine, including headache, nausea, **anorexia,** vomiting, rash, hair loss, and fever. Some researchers believe that the sulfapyridine, although having some beneficial antibacterial qualities, is the reason for the side effects.

Going on this belief, researchers separated the 5-ASA from the compound and used it in enemas, finding it to be at least as beneficial as the sulfasalazine. Other applications soon followed. Here are some of the more common 5-ASA applications used in the treatment of IBD:

Rowasa enemas and Canasa suppositories—These medications involve the introduction of 5-ASA to the mucosa of the rectum (suppository) as well as the sigmoid and descending colon (enema). The suppository, a 500- or 1000-milligram dose—waxy, light tan colored, and bullet shaped—is usually inserted in the rectum one, two, or three times a day, depending on dosage level and response to the drug; the enema comes in a white bottle with a slender tip that is lubricated with white petroleum and contains 4 grams of 5-ASA that is suspended in a milky-colored liquid. The usual dose of the enema is one enema, used at bedtime with the contents held in for eight hours.

The side effects reported with these applications include abdominal pain, rectal pain, nausea, vomiting, gas, hair loss, and headaches. All side effects should be reported to the doctor.

Pentasa and Asacol—These medications use protective coatings to pass the 5-ASA through the upper gastrointestinal tract before releasing it.

Multiple doses of the anti-inflammatory medication must be taken throughout the day to ensure a constant flow of the medication to the mucosa. In Asacol, the brown tablets are coated with a resin that dissolves in the colon where the pH level reaches 7. The usual dose of Asacol is six 400 mg tablets, two taken three times a day; the maintenance dose of Asacol is considered to be two 400 mg tablets taken twice a day; a new formulation of the drug may provide 800 mg per tablet, cutting the number of tablets needed in half. For now, the maximum daily dosage is considered to be four 400 mg tablets taken three times a day. In Pentasa, the medication is contained in microgranules that look like white sprinkles used to decorate cookies and pastries, which are contained in a blue and green capsule in the 250 mg formula, blue only in the 500 mg formula. From the time the capsule passes from the ileum to the colon, the microgranules are slowly dispersed and release the medication onto the ileum and colon. Occasionally, the user of the medication can see the remains of the microgranules in the stool. The dose of this medication to induce remission is four 250 mg tablets or two 500 mg tablets taken four times a day, but it can be effective in some patients in doses of 500 mg taken four times a day.

Lialda—Though this is the same medication as is in Asacol and Pentasa, this medication, approved for use in January 2007, allows the patient to take just one dose of it a day. The tablets, each 1.2 grams, reddish brown, and encased in a film that breaks down in the colon, are taken in doses of two to four pills once a day. They carry the same side effects as the above medications.

The side effects of these medications include abdominal distension, nausea, headaches, hair loss, and dry skin. All side effects should be reported to the doctor.

Colazal and Dipentum—These two medications use substances other than sulfapyridine to cleave to the 5-ASA to protect it from early absorption. In both cases, bacteria in the colon break the bond, releasing the 5-ASA to act on inflammation. In Colazal, each beige 750 mg capsule contains balsalazine disodium that breaks down in the colon to release 5-ASA and an inert substance that is not absorbed by the colon. The usual dose is three 750 mg capsules taken three times a day. The side effects reported in a clinical trial include fatigue, rectal bleeding, gas, and fever. All side effects should be reported to the doctor.

Dipentum uses olsalazine, another 5-ASA molecule, to join with 5-ASA until colonic bacteria break the bond. The doses for Dipentum range from two to four 250 mg tablets, taken three times a day. Logic would dictate that the two 5-ASA chemicals would work double time but that has not proven to be the case as it appears that more water is drawn into the intestines, the major side effect being an unfortunate increase in diarrhea. For this reason, many gastroenterologists at times avoid prescribing this medication.

Steroids

Another age-old group of medications in the treatment of IBD is gluco-corticosteroids. These drugs were first created in 1949 and the common form of prednisone debuted in 1955 as a close synthetic copy of a natural steroid produced in amounts of about 25 mg a day by the outer region of the adrenal gland, located above the kidneys. This natural body chemical is responsible for regulating blood pressure. Of particular interest in IBD, it also helps to control inflammation by altering hormone and cell production and activity, and aides in restoring water and salt balance, leading to better absorption of these items in the intestinal tract.

However, the 25 mg of cortisone is equal to about 5 mg of prednisone. When the inflammation gets out of hand in the intestines, the body needs more cortisone than it can produce, hence the introduction of the medicine. The different forms of the steroids are introduced orally in tablet form and in a delayed release but rapidly metabolized form in foams, creams, and enemas that are topically applied to the anus and rectum and intravenously administered in liquid form for patients with UC and CD.

Prednisone and prednisolone—Perhaps the most commonly used form of this steroid is prednisone. Prednisone is ingested in pill form and the chemicals are taken to the liver where they are converted into prednisolone. During a normal process, the pituitary gland, a master gland in the brain, sends a signal to the adrenal gland to produce natural steroids. When the prednisolone is introduced to the system, the process is interrupted and the adrenal gland production is suppressed. The greater amount of steroids in the body then act to control the inflammatory process and increase the body's ability to absorb water and salt.

Usually, a doctor will prescribe the medication initially at 40 to 60 mg a day, meaning four to six 10 mg small, white pills will be swallowed in a day. As the patient begins to respond to the medication with a lessening of symptoms, the medication is reduced in dosage by 5 to 10 mg every ten days to two weeks.

As the dose drops to below 20 mg, some doctors will decrease the amount of the reduction to 2.5 mg every ten days to two weeks, meaning the person taking the steroid will go from 20 mg one week to 17.5 two weeks later and so on. Occasionally, a doctor will use a pulse technique, meaning the high dose of steroids is initially administered and then dropped quickly, by about 10 mg per day until the dose reaches a more manageable level such as 20 or 10 mg. In either case, the reason for the reduction in the medication is that the adrenal gland needs time to "wake up" and begin producing a normal amount of cortisone again. An immediate termination of the drug may leave the adrenal gland nonfunctioning and result in a drastic drop in blood pressure.

Simply put, the side effects of the drug can be horrendous and can literally affect every part of the body. Common side effects include insomnia, dramatic mood swings, depression, water retention, weight gain, swelling of the face (moon face), development of stretch marks, growth of hair on the body and face, loss of hair on the top of the head, muscle weakness, diabetes, acne, osteoporosis, osteonecrosis, **pancreatitis,** gastritis, and a suppressed immune system. Fortunately, many of the side effects disappear or reverse themselves once the drug is reduced but even the reduction process can bring on changes. People going through steroid withdrawal may suffer from joint pain and depression. Also, some individuals experience a flare of their disease as the amount of the drug is decreased. For these individuals, additional immunosuppressive therapy might be necessary to wean effectively from steroids.

Budesonide—One alternative that individuals with CD from the ileum to the ascending colon have is budesonide (Entocort EC). This drug is enterically coated in a salmon and white 3 mg capsule which breaks apart in the small bowel. It is rapidly metabolized, meaning little of it hangs around in the body to disrupt the adrenal-pituitary connection like prednisone. Its usual dosage is 9 mgs, taken once in the morning, and tapered to 6 mg for two weeks before stopping completely. A maintenance dose of the drug is 6 mg, taken once in the morning. Because it is rapidly metabolized, there are very few side effects associated with Entocort although some individuals may experience increased bruising susceptibility.

Intravenous injectable steroids—At times, people with IBD are not able to take medications by mouth due to an obstruction, severe disease, or surgery. When this happens, cortisone is administered into the muscle by injection or into a vein with an IV drip. There are basically three different kinds of steroids given to people who are already on prednisone: methylprednisone

(SoluMedrol), hydrocortisone (SoluCortef), or prednisolone. The dosage varies on the condition of the patient as well as the amount the patient was taking before being admitted to the hospital. The side effects of the IV or injected steroids are the same as the oral steroids.

In individuals who are not currently on steroids, a synthetic hormone, adrenocorticotropic hormone (ACTH), used to stimulate the adrenal gland into producing more natural cortisone is given to the patient. In the case of Entocort, prescribing information suggests that care be taken in introducing systemic steroids and not stopping them immediately, but rather slowly weaning the individual.

Enemas and other topical steroids—In cases where the individuals have ulcerative proctitis, left-sided ulcerative colitis, or CD in the rectum, sigmoid, or descending colon, suppositories, enemas, and foams can be used like similar 5-ASA preparations to reduce the inflammation. Unlike the 5-ASA preparations, varying levels of the hydrocortisone in the preparations are absorbed into the body and can act like the ingested forms of steroids.

With the foam, an aerosol container filled with foam is included in a package with a small white applicator. With Cortifoam, the foamy, white medicine is drawn off the container and into the applicator, which is then inserted into the anus and the contents slowly pushed into the anus. The relief is almost immediate and feels almost cooling to the inflamed area. Each application delivers about 80 milligrams of hydrocortisone and is used once or twice a day, every day for two to three weeks and then every other day for two weeks before stopping. ProctoFoam is basically the same in application and effect.

Cortenema is a hydrocortisone enema, much like the Rowasa enema in design and application but with the steroid as the active ingredient; the usual dose is one 60 mL enema (100 mg hydrocortisone) daily, though some use them twice a day. Like the hydrocortisone foams, the nightly enemas are effective for a short time and are weaned within a month of starting them. Side effects of these medications are similar to the oral steroids but include a rash and rectal pain. A Proctocort suppository contains 30 mg of hydrocortisone in a bullet-shaped waxy form. It is inserted into the rectum two or three times a day for two weeks.

Hydrocortisone creams such as the over the counter Anusol HC (with one percent or less of hydrocortisone) or the prescription strength Proctocort Cream (with 1 percent hydrocortisone) or Proctozone HC (with 2.5

percent hydrocortisone) are helpful in reducing anal itching and to shrink inflamed hemorrhoidal tissues. These soothing creams are applied after wiping following a bowel movement and provide relief in minutes. A thin film can be applied directly to the anal opening or a small amount can be applied within about the first half inch of the anal canal with a small applicator. Other than a potential for a rash, these medications have few side effects.

Immunomodulators

The theory behind using medication to suppress the immune system is that a lessened immune system will have a diminished capacity to cause harm in the intestines. The few drugs used the most in this capacity were initially created not for IBD but to treat childhood leukemia and adult cancers, and to discourage the immune systems of transplant patients from attacking the implanted donor organ.

Azathioprine and 6-mercaptopurine—Azathioprine (Imuran, Azasan) and its close cousin, 6-mercaptopurine (Purinethol), are the most commonly used immunosuppressives in IBD therapy in both UC and CD patients though no one is really sure exactly the effect these drugs have, whether immunosuppressive or anti-inflammatory. What is known is that white cell production is slowed, leading to less potential for inflammation. Purinethol comes in 50 mg scored white tablets, Imuran comes in 50 mg scored yellow to off-white tablets, and Azasan comes in 75 mg scored yellow triangular tablets and 100 mg scored yellow diamond-shaped tablets. All of these can be broken at the score mark for half doses. The dose of the drug depends on the individual; some people can achieve remission on as little as 12.5 mg of the drug while others only begin to see a reduction of symptoms at dosages that exceed 100 mg.

The effects of the drug usually kick in anywhere from a few weeks to six months after beginning the medication. After beginning the medication, the patient will have to have blood drawn on a schedule that starts weekly for a month, every other week for two months and every other month for the duration of the time that the patient is on the drug. Using the blood tests, the physician can check for dangerously low levels of white blood cells, a condition called leukopenia; low platelet levels, a condition called thrombocytopenia; anemia; or low hemoglobin levels, as well as abnormal levels of liver enzymes. These conditions are reversed with the withdrawal of the medication.

Tests in a handful of U.S. labs have been developed in the past decade to measure a certain metabolite called 6-tg or 6-thioguanine, in addition to a particular enzyme that is needed to metabolize the drug in the first place. These tests provide a good target for a therapeutic range for the drugs, reducing the chance of ingesting overly effective levels, potentially resulting in liver damage.

Side effects of 6-MP and azathioprine include nausea, fever, rash, joint pain, and the dangerous blood level suppression mentioned before. Small numbers of patients on the drugs may suffer pancreatitis while even smaller patient populations have reported certain lymphomas.

Methotrexate—Methotrexate is gaining acceptability as an alternative or companion medication of 6-MP and azathioprine. Originally used to treat certain cancers, "metho," as it is perhaps more popularly known in the patient population, acts to slow the production of rapidly reproducing cells. Although it is used as an oral medication in other chronic diseases like psoriasis and rheumatoid arthritis, it is injected into the muscles of IBD patients, usually in a 25 mg dose. A majority of patients participating in a number of smaller trials were initially successful in achieving remission in the early months of the trials, but a varying number were unable to maintain that remission at one year.

Some of the side effects of methotrexate include hair loss and inflammation in the mouth. Although patients with psoriasis and to a lesser extent rheumatoid arthritis at times have scarring in the liver, that is not usually seen in IBD patients.

Cyclosporine—Cyclosporine (Sandimmune, Neoral) was first invented in the 1980s and its use caused the world of transplantation to increase success rates. Since that time, the potent, rapidly acting immunosuppressant drug has been used in the treatment of a variety of illnesses, including some like IBD that require immunosuppression. In IBD, it has found its greatest success in the short-term usage in individuals who are severely ill with IBD and in individuals with CD who cannot take the other immunomodulatory medications due to allergy.

Cyclosporine comes in soft gel capsules and in a solution that can be mixed with milk or orange juice; for individuals who can't tolerate taking oral medication, it can be injected or placed in an IV drip. The most serious side effects of the drug are the seizures that occur in some patients and the damage that can occur to the kidneys, both acutely and chronically.

Tacrolimus—Tacrolimus (Prograf) was studied in the late 1990s and early 2000s as an immunomodulator for use in CD and UC but had already been approved for use in post-transplant patients for immunosuppression. This drug has been shown to be effective in treating severe forms of IBD, as it is rapidly acting and because it serves as a good substitute for those who can't tolerate the other immunosuppressives. Though it is commonly used in .5 mg (light yellow), 1 mg (white) or 5 mg (grayish-red) capsules, it also comes in a topical cream that has been shown in studies to be effective in treating CD in the mouth and the perianal area, as well as effective in healing enterocutaneous fistulas; it is also used in IBD patients with the extraintestinal manifestation pyoderma gangrenosum.

Like all immunosuppressives, tacrolimus carries with it a host of potentially dangerous side effects, including tremor, headache, diarrhea, hypertension, nausea, vomiting, and abnormal renal function. It also can interact with a number of medications, so it is important for the prescribing physician to be aware of every medication taken, not only those for IBD.

Biologic drugs

When I wrote about biologic medication in the first edition five years ago, these drugs were brand new to the marketplace, so new that only one had been approved for use and only in adults with CD with severe or fistulaszing disease. Since that time, extensive study has taken place, producing the probable approval of two new drugs this year and several more probably coming to the market in the next few years. Biologic medications are now used in tens of thousands of CD and UC patients, in children and adults. Additionally, a lot more is known about the risks of such medication, as well as about the dosing.

To understand how these medications work, it is important to grasp the role of different cells in the inflammatory process. Inflammation occurs when certain cells send out signals to other cells that an action is needed. The intended cells receive that message and signal to a few other types of cells the same message, and so on. Try to picture dominoes standing on end in a chain reaction, with a single line branching off and then further branching off. When the first domino falls, the others rapidly follow suit. But if you remove a few of the dominoes, the destruction can be contained.

That is the same theory used in biologic therapy. If we can stop the cells from communicating their messages or stop them from producing in the first place, we short-circuit that process and stop the destruction before it starts. Cells that either increase or decrease inflammatory activity in the body include tumor necrosis factor alpha, a number of interleukins, alpha 4 integrin, intercellular adhesion molecules, and interferon gamma. The goal of biologic therapy is to disrupt these cells' activities by binding to them or inhibiting their production, the result of which is to stop that chain reaction before it starts and preventing the inflammatory process. Because their actions are so specific in that they only affect certain cells, these drugs theoretically are more desirable than the immunosuppressives and steroids that are broader in their cellular suppression abilities.

In the case of tumor necrosis factor alpha (TNF-alpha), the body produces this cytokine in abundance in people with certain kinds of autoimmune conditions, including CD, UC, rheumatoid arthritis, psoriasis, and ankylosing spondylitis. In CD and UC, TNF-alpha has been found in abundance in the blood and feces of patients who are flaring. Infliximab (Remicade) was the first anti–TNF-alpha drug to be released. Made of 25 percent mouse component and 75 percent human component, the drug is infused into a patient's arm over a few hours; it quickly binds with the TNF-alpha and prevents it from starting up the inflammatory chain reaction. When it appeared in 1999, Remicade initially was prescribed to help close fistulas (with doses at week zero, week two, and week six) or to induce and maintain remission, given in eight-week intervals and usually in tandem with 6-MP, azathioprine, or methotrexate.

Since that time, we have learned that some people who were given this drug developed tuberculosis, likely from a latent infection that became active due to a suppressed immune system. Because of this, those who are prescribed this therapy must undergo tuberculosis testing prior to the first infusion. Further, recent studies indicate that there may be an increase in the number of cancers, including lymphoma and skin cancers, among those who use these anti–TNF-alpha drugs; however, the evidence is hardly definitive, as those who use the drugs have naturally higher rates of lymphomas anyway, and the skin cancer rates were not significantly higher than appeared in the general population.

In 2006, Remicade was approved for use in UC in both adults and children. It is given on the same dosing schedule as it was for CD, but some individuals require more of the drug either at the time of infusion or at intervals that are as close as five weeks apart. The effective dose and schedule is a very individual aspect of this treatment and should be determined by the doctor prescribing it.

The drug is usually administered in a hospital or in an infusion room at a physician's office. The dose is initially based on the patient's weight and is usually administered through a vein in the arm. Many infusion settings require the patient to stay for a short period of time after the infusion is complete to allow the physician to monitor for and treat any possible allergic reactions.

In 2007, two more anti–TNF-alpha drugs will likely be approved for use in treating CD, as both performed well in phase III testing. Adalimumab (Humira), the first fully humanized anti–TNF-alpha drug, has already been approved for use in RA, ankylosing spondylitis, and psoriatic arthritis. After undergoing tuberculosis testing, patients in its trials were given anywhere from 80 mg to 160 mg in subcutaneous injections for the first week, with 40 mg injections every week or every other week thereafter. Many also used immunosuppressive drugs to enter remission and remain there. Certolizumab pegol (Cimzia) is a new drug; it has not been approved for other uses, as Humira and Remicade both have. It has about five percent mouse component and 95 percent human. Also a subcutaneous injection, it was given in a loading dose of 400 mg at weeks zero, two, and four, and then every four weeks after that, achieving remission in most study participants.

Natalizumab (Tysabri), an alpha 4 integrin inhibitor, also performed very well in studies of CD patients. The infusion drug is typically given in 300 mg doses through an IV over the space of an hour, once every four weeks. The drug was previously approved for use in MS patients, but clinical trials were halted at one point because two MS patients and one CD patient contracted a rare viral infection, progressive multifocal leukoencephalopathy (PML), which usually leads to death or disability; one MS patient and the CD patient died of the infection. The complication appeared to have occurred in those who were either recently exposed to immunosuppressants or who were taking the drugs at the time the virus was discovered. Because of this, those who are infused with the drug have to take their treatment at an approved infusion center. The drug has not yet been approved for CD but is a likely candidate for that step in the coming months.

Sargamostim (Leukine), a granulocyte macrophage colony stimulating factor, was originally developed as a leukemia drug. It helped patients recover from chemotherapy by promoting the production of two key white cells, thereby helping them avoid potentially life threatening fungal infections when their immune systems were down. Now, you may ask, what would a CD patient be doing taking a drug like this, one that stimulates the immune system rather than suppressing it? It's a fair question. It has to do with a theory that suggests that CD occurs in people with defective, under-performing immune systems, which could possibly be helped by the production of specific white cells.

Two more biologic drugs entered the final phase of testing immediately prior to the publication of this book are Orencia (abatacept) and Prochymal (adult mesenchymal stem cells). Abatacept blocks a chemical that causes the T-cells to become active, a step that is a little earlier in the inflammatory cycle than the current anti–TNF-alpha drugs work. The drug is currently approved for use in rheumatoid arthritis and is being tested in both UC and CD. It is administered intravenously in an infusion center setting.

Prochymal is being tested in both CD and acute graft versus host disease (GvHD), an inflammatory condition found in post-stem cell transplant patients; GvHD is similar to CD in that the newly transplanted immune system turns on certain body parts and attacks them. This product, which will likely be approved within the next year or two, relies on mesenchymal stem cells to slow down production of TNF-alpha and interferon-gamma, another pro-inflammatory cytokine; the stem cells are harvested from the marrow of healthy adult donors. Additionally, Prochymal may also help to repair tissue damaged in the inflammatory process. Prochymal is administered via intravenous infusion.

In a report that appeared in the *New England Journal of Medicine* in 2005, patients receiving the drug did not achieve remission in statistically greater rates than those receiving placebo, but it did help reduce disease activity in those receiving the drug. Studies are continuing.

A number of other drugs are currently being developed and tested as biologic therapies for both CD and UC. For example, alicaforsen has been performing well in phase II studies of UC patients. This drug, used as a

240 mg enema, inhibits production of intercellular adhesion molecules (ICAM-1) that multiply in UC patients during a flare-up. The drug initially was tested as an infusion drug in CD patients but was not found to be efficacious in inducing and maintaining remission. Fontolizumab (HuZAF), an anti-interferon gamma infusion drug, did well in early trials for CD patients. Visilizumab (Nuvion) is in trials for both CD and UC. These and more drugs will likely be making headlines in the months and years to come as they progress through trial phases.

Antibiotics

In IBD, infections can happen at any time. There are the infections that occur in CD when the bowel wall is breached and an abscess forms; in UC, peritonitis can occur with perforation resulting from toxic megacolon. Because of these instances and others, the use of antibiotics may be unavoidable in many patients.

Metronidazole and ciprofloxacin—The use of antibiotics as a mainline treatment of IBD is not entirely uncommon and may be used for some cases of CD of the colon. In that case metronidazole (Flagyl) is used starting in 250 mg doses that are increased slowly until symptoms subside, usually in two to four months, and then weaned after about six months. The side effects of the treatment, outside of the terrible metallic taste the generic form of the pills can leave in the mouth, include peripheral neuropathy, a tingling sensation in the hands and feet. The side effect disappears in most cases as soon as the drug is withdrawn.

Metronidazole is also used alone to treat perianal CD and in combination with another antibiotic, ciprofloxacin (Cipro), to clear up abscesses in CD. In the case of perforation due to toxic megacolon in UC patients, intravenous medications are usually administered until the threat of infection passes, at which time they are withdrawn.

Another drug, rifaximin (Xifaxan), is a nonabsorbed antibiotic used to treat traveler's diarrhea. Instead of working through the blood to kill bacteria, it works directly to clean out the undesirable bacteria from the lumen, the hollow space of the intestines. Some small studies have found it to be helpful in CD patients, while it is also being studied for use in UC, specifically for use in pouchitis. Further studies are needed.

Other investigational drugs and treatments

A number of drug therapies are being studied at this time for the treatment of CD or UC or both. To name them all would be impossible. However, those that target specific inflammatory cell interactions and functions are practically multiplying, while development of other drugs and therapies continues to move along at a seemingly rapid pace. To find out how the drug trials function, see Month 11.

This is an interesting time for other medical therapies to be developed as well. Currently, three potential CD therapies appear promising. It is important to note that they are all still in the testing process and won't be available with FDA approval for a few years, if at all.

The first, autologous stem cell transplant, involves rounds of chemotherapy to knock out the bone marrow and then an infusion of the patient's own stem cells, creating a sort of resetting of the immune system. That therapy is in phase II testing in the United States. For the most part, patients from the first phase of testing appear not to have had the disease return following transplant.

Another therapy, now in phase III testing, is the Adacolumn Apheresis system. In this nifty bit of technology, a patient's blood is filtered of certain white cells that are excessive in the blood of CD patients; the filtered blood is then returned to the body. The results of the study will likely be available within the next two years.

A third therapy is based on the theory that the people with IBD are missing an antigen which turns the immune system against the body. By creating medicine from proteins found in the patient's own colon, the researchers were able to force the disease into remission in a remarkable percentage of study subjects. The technology is currently in phase II testing in Israel.

IN A SENTENCE:

> Although there is no current cure for IBD, there is a veritable arsenal of medications to treat the diseases.

living

Living with the Effects of Medication

SOME WOULD say the treatment is worse than the disease. And at times, I would have to agree. I, along with many of the individuals you have already learned from in this book, have suffered everything from sepsis to sore joints, from hair loss to hairy tongues.

Really, what is the choice? You can take the medication, reduce the symptoms, and learn to live with the side effects, or you can not take the medication, suffer terribly, and perhaps succumb to an obstruction, a perforation, or a bacterial infection. Not much of a choice, is it?

Side effects to live with

Perhaps the side effects that people complain about the most have to do with that nasty drug, prednisone. On prednisone, your body may change shape completely, whether you do something about it or not. One reason for this is that fat distribution in the body changes and tends to collect more in areas such as the stomach, the face, and on the back of the neck. As stated before, steroids help to improve the efficiency of the body's ability to handle water and salt. Because of this, you may notice that water tends to collect in your joints or other areas, sometimes so badly that you can press the affected area of the body and leave an indentation. Another reason for the body changes has to do with the ravenous hunger you may be feeling all of the time. The hunger gets so intense that you may find yourself barely finishing one meal before you are eagerly planning your next.

Believe it or not, there is a little good news with the body changes. For one, the changes are temporary and reversible with the withdrawal of the medication. For another, there are some minor alterations you can make in your lifestyle to help control some of the changes.

Dietary changes for people on prednisone fall more on the side of logical rather than proven by a multicenter, double blind, placebo-controlled study. For example, if you are hungry all the time, eat smaller meals more frequently. If you wait too long, your hunger may be uncontrollable and you will crave easily accessible junk food rather than something healthy such as a banana or a baked yam. Make sure you pitch all your junk food and stock up on healthy, easy to prepare snack choices such as salt-free pretzels and graham crackers. Have bananas or water-packed canned fruit when you can't help but give in to cravings.

Another change is to switch to a low fat, low sodium diet. Sodium helps us to retain water while fat can accumulate more readily. If water retention gets out of hand and you find your fingers, toes, ankles, and any other joint swelling, eat more natural diuretics like licorice, watermelon, or asparagus, or ask your doctor about taking a diuretic such as Lasix. Beware that you will have to urinate more while on these medications, but they can help to relieve some of the bloated feeling.

Yet another area that can be helped with dietary changes has to do with the onset of osteoporosis, the increase in porosity caused by bone loss that is usually related to aging, but is common in individuals with long-term steroid usage or disease activity. The problem with increasing the dietary intake of calcium-containing dairy products is that it means consuming more of the milk-based sugar lactose, a difficult proposition for individuals with IBD who are more likely to be **lactose intolerant** than the general population. In recent years, more and more food companies have been enriching their foods with calcium citrate, an easily absorbed form of the mineral. Bread, cereals, fruit juices, waffles, and hundreds of other food products contain this bone-building mineral. If you still are not able to incorporate these foods into your diet, talk to your doctor about adding a daily calcium supplement to your regimen. While you are at it, try to eliminate some bone-leaching things from your diet like coffee, tea, and soda pop.

Insomnia is a common side effect felt by individuals taking steroids, which also thankfully goes away as the drug is tapered. Even knowing this, it is difficult to endure as you stare at the ceiling, praying for the wings of Morpheus to take you to your dreams. The lack of sleep the next day registers as lethargy and crankiness, not good qualities most especially if you work, study, or live with others. One way to combat this is to get to sleep early. If you usually don't climb under the covers until Letterman signs off, try hitting the hay as early as 8:30 P.M. By doing this, you are sure to get a decent amount of sleep, even if you are awake for three hours until you fall asleep. The extra rest will help, as you require more rest during illness and recovery. If this change is impossible, talk to your doctor about trying a mild over-the-counter, nonaddictive sleep aid such as Tylenol PM, Sominex, or a mild prescription medication such as Restoril or Xanax.

Getting extra rest may help with the mood swings you might experience on the medication but even with the extra sleep, mood swings are tough to cope with. The good part about them are the manias. During these excessively happy times, you will feel more aware, more capable, more energetic than you have ever felt in your life. But then comes the bad part of the swings, the deep dark depression that sends you into crying fits and jags and an outlook on life that is bleak at best. First of all, realize that this, too, shall pass as the medication is weaned. Second, give yourself room to feel the feelings and ask for patience from others who will find you difficult to deal with at best sometimes. Third, seek help from a psychotherapist during this time if you think it will help (information on finding a psychotherapist can be found in Day 4). In particular, you may ask your physician about a psychotropic medication that will help to stabilize your mood.

Skin and hair changes are also difficult but can be managed. Utilizing a regular skin care regimen and avoiding fatty foods, for example, can avert acne. Stretch marks due to thinning skin are permanent scars but can be reduced by using certain prescription preparations such as tretinoin cream or by rubbing the insides of vitamin E capsules on the affected area. After the medication is withdrawn, certain laser procedures may help reduce the appearance of stretch marks as well. A dermatologist can be particularly helpful during this time.

As for the body hair, sometimes there is just no avoiding these effects. Facial and body hair growth can be excessive in some people but barely noticeable in others. There are prescription creams and over the counter depilatory lotions that can be rubbed on the skin to discourage hair growth; again, a dermatologist can help with this. Some people have no luck, no matter what they do. In this case, it helps to develop a personal strategy to cope. One female patient I met while covering a story on heart transplants found that the steroids caused such excessive hair growth on her face that the only way to deal with it was to shave twice a day. While most women would cringe at the thought, this trooper was just happy that there was a way for her to deal with the change.

For head hair, there is little to do when it begins to fall from your head. Again, developing a personal strategy is the key. Hats and scarves work for some, while others with more serious hair loss may find cover in a wig. When I was on prednisone the last time, I gained twenty-five pounds in no time, my face blew up into the shape of the moon, my fingers looked and felt like sausages, and my moods went up and down more often than a car on a roller coaster. On one particular morning, I looked into the mirror after a shower and noticed that my hair was thinner than ever. Large amounts of it were stuck in the drain and on the towel I used to dry it with. It was more than I could take. After I finished a good cry, I marched off to the hairdresser and ordered him to cut it short. The short, sexy haircut he gave me hid the thinning hair and gave me a quick boost in self-esteem I so desperately needed at that point.

Another major side effect to worry about is shared by immunosuppressives, biologics, and steroids—suppressed immune function and the related increased susceptibility to infection. This effect occurs because all three drug classes act to suppress at least one area of the immune system, thus rendering it unable or less effective to fight off bacterial, viral, or fungal infections.

A compromised immune system makes you susceptible to every cold and throat infection that happens your way. And the illnesses will tend to last longer and be worse than you ever remember them being. To ward these sicknesses off, use your common sense. Be sure to maintain proper nutrition and to get adequate rest. Practice good hygiene, washing your hands often in warm, soapy water for at least twenty seconds before rinsing (sing the alphabet song once or Row, Row, Row Your Boat three times for the proper amount of time). Avoid touching your eyes, nose, and mouth with unwashed hands. Tell all of your friends and relatives to inform you of anyone who is ill prior to attending any gatherings of family or friends. Be especially vigilant in avoiding anyone who has or may have the chicken pox, even if you have had the virus in the past; exposure to the virus may lead to an occurrence of shingles, a nasty, painful condition related to the chicken pox virus. Get the flu shot in October. Avoid crowded areas like the shopping mall or football stadiums during the flu season. If you should get sick, be aware of your symptoms and report any fever to your doctor, as it may be indicative of disease activity.

Thrush is a special illness I'd like to single out because its occurrence is not rare in immune-suppressed patients. Thrush is an overgrowth of a fungus known as candida albicans that commonly appears as a whitish film on the tongue and occasionally spreads into the throat. At times, the film is accompanied by sores on the tongue, in the cheek, or in the throat that can be painful. This fungus is also responsible for vaginal yeast infections in women and in the type of thrush that babies get in their mouths or diaper areas. Doctors usually prescribe a mouthwash with nystatin or other similar antifungal medications to eliminate the infection and suggest that gentle brushing of the affected area can help while warm, salt-water rinses can ease the pain. It usually disappears within two weeks with treatment.

Side effects to report

Occasionally, a medication we take can cause allergic side effects or we can be so sensitive to the medication that even a small dose can cause major effects. Our liver or kidneys may also bear the brunt too greatly. In any case, some side effects will occur and should be reported immediately to your doctor, including:

- Strong pain in the joints, making them feel as if they are broken or immobile
- Tingling in your hands and feet
- Dizziness or fainting
- Chills or sweating
- Difficulty breathing or feeling as if your throat is closing
- Swelling of your lips, tongue, or face

○ Appearance of hives
○ Severe worsening of symptoms such as fever, abdominal pain, bloody diarrhea, or vomiting
○ Pale stools or dark urine
○ Painful or difficult urination
○ Severe headache or blurred vision
○ Appearance of pink or purple dots on the skin

IN A SENTENCE:

> The side effects of the medication to treat IBD can be brutal, but they can be managed if you have a coping plan in place.

Drugs That Help, Drugs That Hurt

AS YOU have just learned in the last week, there are scads of medicines out there to help ease inflammation by controlling the inflammatory process in one way or another. These pills, creams, injections, infusions, lotions, enemas, foams, and suppositories help patients to quell or quiet the disease activity and are necessary for survival in some cases.

However, there is another set of drugs—both prescription and over the counter medications—that help patients alleviate daily diarrhea, nausea, painful spasms, bone loss, and depression. These medications that help us to live a close proximity to a normal life are called supportive therapies.

While all of these helpful medications exist, yet another set of drugs have the potential to do the opposite, possibly sending us right back into relapse. Nonsteroidal anti-inflammatory drugs (NSAIDs), antibiotics, and others can cause symptoms to flare in some individuals with IBD. From now on, you should discuss the use of any of these medications thoroughly with your doctor before using them.

Drugs that help

Supportive medication in IBD plays a role that can be just as important as the different classes of anti-inflammatory medication that are considered the main treatments for CD and UC. These medications include antidiarrhea, antispasmodic, antinausea, antidepressant, and biphosphonate drugs.

Antidiarrheal medication—As the name suggests, these medications reduce the occurrence of diarrhea, one of the main, shared symptoms of UC and CD. For the most part, the drugs, whether narcotic or not, act to slow the intestine's neuromotor responses, which in turn reduces crampy, urgent feelings in the rectum and the number of bowel movements.

Loperamide (Imodium), an over the counter medication, is usually tried first, using one or two pills after a bowel movement and one after each subsequent bowel movement until the diarrhea stops for a while. Atropine with diphenoxylate (Lomotil) combines the antispasmodic effects of atropine and the antidiarrhea effects of diphenoxylate to reduce diarrhea activity. Deodorized tincture of opium, paregoric (containing powdered opium), hydrocodone, and codeine are all opiates and work to slow intestinal movements; all also carry a chance of addiction as they are narcotics.

One other antidiarrheal medication, cholestyramine (Questran), was approved originally as a drug to lower blood cholesterol levels. Helpful to CD patients with ileal disease or resection, it acts to bind with bile acids that are normally reabsorbed in healthy ileums. Unbound bile acids cause more water to enter the colon, resulting in more diarrhea; the powdered medication, taken one to three times a day and mixed with juice, helps to avoid this situation.

A strong note of caution is important in using antidiarrheal medication in patients who have severe UC and CD as they may herald the onset of toxic megacolon.

Antispasmodic medication—These little powerhouses can stop an attack of intestinal spasms in their tracks before they have a chance to get started. These medications are also helpful to individuals with functional bowel diseases such as irritable bowel syndrome (IBS), a condition that may coexist in many IBD patients.

Mostly taken by pill or a pill placed under the tongue to dissolve (sublingual), these medications—including dicyclomine hydrochloride (Bentyl), hyoscamine (Levsin), propantheline (Pro-Banthine, also used to treat excessive secretions), and belladonna alkaloids with phenobarbitol (Donnatol)—help regulate the neuromotor activity affecting the intestinal muscles. Often times, a patient has to try at least a couple of these drugs to find one that works on his or her symptoms.

All of these medications can cause sleepiness, affect muscle coordination, and are contraindicated with alcohol use. Side effects also include dry mouth. Again, these medications are contraindicated in individuals where toxic megacolon is a concern. In general, they should not be used with the antidiarrheal drugs previously mentioned.

Antinausea medication—Usually, nausea and vomiting in IBD indicate disease activity or are the result of a side effect of medication. Because of this, nausea and vomiting, however unpleasant, are useful in letting a physician know that there is something about which to be concerned.

At other times, nausea and vomiting are nuisances with which we must learn to cope. One coping method is the use of antinausea medication. Prochlorperazine (Compazine), promethazine (Phenergan), trimethobenzamide (Tigan), and ondansetron HCl (Zofran) are all commonly prescribed oral antinausea medications. The drugs carry different side effects, have different medication interactions, and come in different dosages and other forms. It is important for your physician to know exactly what you are taking in terms of both over the counter and prescription medication.

Antidepressant medication—Let it be said again that there is no psychological syndrome or profile associated with either CD or UC. However, as detailed in earlier chapters, the uncertainty that often accompanies chronic illness can lead to depression. Also, it has been noted in at least one small study that a bout with depression often precedes disease activity in people with UC. Because of this, some patients may find relief through the use of antidepressant medication such as Wellbutrin, Elavil, or Prozac, to name a few.

Biphosphonates and other bone-building drugs—Because bone loss can happen with both CD and UC, it makes sense that one of the therapies prescribed at times to IBD patients is targeted at protecting or rebuilding bone density. For this reason, doctors prescribe biphosphonates and other bone-building medications to prevent or slow the mechanism associated with bone loss.

As stated on page 79, the bone-building process involves both bone resorption and bone formation. When this process is interrupted, bones become less dense and therefore less strong. The goal of bone-building medications is to change this process, allowing more formation activity, less resorption, and potentially stronger bones.

Biphosphonates are a class of drugs that slow the resorptive process, allowing for increased bone formation. Alendronate sodium (Fosamax) and risendronate sodium (Actonel) are available in tablets taken daily or weekly, while ibandronate sodium (Boniva) can be taken once a month as a pill or four times a year as an infusion. The side effects of the medications include heartburn, nausea, and headache.

Other drugs used in the bone-building process are more hormonally based and generally used in menopausal women, those who tend to have the highest risk of osteoporosis-related fractures. Estrogen therapy and hormonal therapy are commonly prescribed in this population, as is calcitonin, a hormone that regulates the level of calcium, which tends to decrease as women age. Women of this age should talk to their doctors about these therapies and which is right for them. One other hormonal therapy, teriparatide (Forteo), increases bone formation and thus density. It comes in a daily injection to be taken for two years and was approved for use in men and women.

One thing IBD patients should know about these drugs is that, by and large, they were not tested in young-adult populations, since osteoporosis and osteopenia tend to be conditions affecting older adults. Because of this, patients should carefully weigh their options, with their doctor's input, before starting on these medications.

Drugs that hurt

Not all anti-inflammatory medications were created equal. Some, like prednisone, Entocort, or the 5-ASA drugs, work well in controlling intestinal inflammation through various means. Others can wreak havoc on the intestines, causing bleeding in individuals who don't have IBD and causing those who do have the diseases to have a flareup or experience a worsening of symptoms.

On the surface, nonsteroidal anti-inflammatory drugs (NSAIDs) would seem like a good thing. Think about it. All of the anti-inflammatory power without the yucky side effects of a steroid, right? Wrong. While these drugs inhibit inflammation by blocking some of the cellular reactions, they also carry the nasty side effect of increased bleeding in the stomach and the intestines. This is because the action of the medication causes the repression of an enzyme called Cyclooxegenase-1 (COX-1), which acts to protect the stomach lining; another enzyme, the pain-causing COX-2, is also repressed. In particular, numerous case studies have linked an increase in symptoms or a flareup of disease in patients with IBD. The names of these drugs include ibuprofen (Advil, Motrin), aspirin (Anacin, Ascriptin, Bayer, Bufferin, Ecotrin), naproxen sodium (Aleve), and ketoprofen (Orudis). One exception to this is the use of baby aspirin (81 mg dose) to prevent blood clots or heart disease in those who are susceptible.

Another new kind of anti-inflammatory medication, COX-2 inhibitors, debuted in recent years; they promise to deliver the power to reduce swelling without compromising the stomach since COX-1 is not repressed. While this is a fantastic development in those with rheumatoid arthritis who can't take NSAIDs because of stomach bleeding, there have been no large studies done on the safety and efficacy of the drug in individuals with IBD; one small study is under way in Pennsylvania regarding the safety of celeoxib (Celebrex) in CD patients, the results of which may soon be available. There have been other small studies that have found a reason to avoid the drugs, including one in which rats with induced colitis had an increase in inflammation while on the drugs. And there have been other papers that theorize a possible treatment for UC or Crohn's colitis who have abnormal levels of COX-2 in their colons. But there have been no long-term large studies on these drugs and their effect on IBD. For that reason alone, you should talk to your doctor about using these medications before ingesting them.

Certain antibiotics definitely have a role in treating CD and UC. The benefits are seen in their ability to clear up abscesses and to improve perianal disease. However, in some individuals, the use of antibiotics has been known to precede cases of clostridium difficile, a condition that causes colitis-like symptoms. This condition happens because the normal gastrointestinal flora balance is suppressed with antibiotic therapy, allowing an environment where the bacterium can multiply in great numbers. The bacteria then release a toxin that causes the ulceration and inflammation. The inflammation is known as **pseudomembranous colitis.**

It is possible that this inflammation can lead to a flareup or worsening of symptoms of IBD in the colon. For this reason, it is very important to discuss the use of antibiotics with your physician before embarking on a treatment program.

IN A SENTENCE:

> Knowing which supportive therapies are available can be a comfort, and realizing which medications can cause harm can help you to avoid unpleasant flare-ups.

living

Compliance

LIVING WITH any chronic illness forces affected individuals to change their perception of what is "normal." With CD and UC, this is no different. You probably scout out the bathroom locations in any public place before you take your coat off now, whereas you never did before. You may become more familiar with medical terms and functions of your intestines whereas before you wouldn't give a hoot. You have changed, and therefore you priorities have changed as well.

One major change you have likely experienced at this point is taking medication on a daily basis. In the past, you may have been prescribed a medication for an infection for ten days to two weeks at the most. Sure, the medication was a hassle to take but you probably felt better when you finished it. And when you were done you returned to a medication-free lifestyle. There was a defined amount of time for you to be taking medication, a payoff, and the resumption of normal activity.

With the disease, you probably juggle taking multiple medications at various times of the day, an annoying task at best. There will be monthly trips to the drugstore to coordinate refills on medication and coinciding trips or calls to the doctor to obtain the refill prescriptions. And you likely will contend with your feelings about taking medication. While some people don't mind taking the medication, others see it as a constant reminder that they have an illness.

But being compliant with medication orders is very important, not only for IBD but for all diseases. Recent studies have shown that noncompliance with medication leads to 125,000 deaths annually in the United States and is a factor in 10 percent of all hospital admissions. In IBD, the 5-ASA drugs we take are separated by hours to provide a constant flow of the anti-inflammatory medication to the mucosa; the prednisone pills should be taken regularly with a slowly tapering dose to allow the adrenal gland to resume normal functions; and the immunosuppressive medication should be taken daily to maintain a suppressed immune system. While missing any one dose of these medications is not going to spell disaster, regularly missing doses will likely make the effect of the drug less and your symptoms greater. So, by the end of this week, do something good and promise yourself that you will come up with a good strategy to become compliant with your medication.

Finding the time and place

One way to make it easier to remember your pills is to take your medication around mealtimes and bedtime. Few of us like to skip meals and all of us have to sleep so this makes it an ideal way to remember. If you use a day planner, write in the times to take medication and keep handy a list of medication that has to be taken and at what times. If you are particularly bad at remembering your medication, employ others to help you through phone calls or gentle reminders.

Making sure your medication is visible is also an easy way to remember to take it. Although you should always use care with medication around children, stashing the bottles in a drawer or a cupboard leaves them out of sight and out of mind. Jerri finds she is best able to remember her medication by leaving it out on the counter in her kitchen, a place she often visits during the day. "I know what it means to have to swallow hordes of pills daily and I don't really enjoy that too much. But who really does?" she said. "While at home I would keep all of the bottles out in the open so there is a constant reminder."

Ordering medication from the pharmacy is yet another thing to be remembered. If you can, coordinate the refills so that you only make

How to give yourself a shot

In the past, medications for CD and UC required only placing the tablet in your mouth and washing it down with a glass of water. But the newer biologic medications have yet to be developed in a pill form and require either an infusion in a clinical setting or the administration of a subcutaneous injection. Although methotrexate is available in pill form, it is usually prescribed as an injection.

Giving yourself a shot can be a very scary thing, especially for needle-phobic people like me. But with preparation and practice, it becomes a whole lot easier than going to the doctor and having a nurse do it for you. That said, learning the process from a health care provider like a doctor or a nurse is the essential first step. When I was learning to give myself shots, Rita, the physician's assistant in my gastroenterologist's office, worked with me for months, first to give me the shots, then to teach me to do it, and finally to walk me through it so I could do it on my own. Without her patient and thorough instruction, I would still be heading to the doctor's office every week for the shot instead of doing it on my own.

When giving yourself a shot, the key to confidence and to technique is to make sure that you have everything you need within easy reach. For this reason, it may be helpful to choose a place where a clean, clear, sturdy surface is within a foot or two of where you will be sitting. I usually choose the nightstand next to my bed or the counter in my bathroom. Wherever you choose, lay out what you will need, first making sure the surface is clean. The shots used currently in biologic therapies come in preloaded syringes, which in turn are packaged in sealed plastic trays; alcohol swabs are provided in the packaging. Check the date on the packaging to make sure the medication hasn't expired; don't use it if it has. Unwrap the package and keep the needle in the tray with the cap on while you gather a cotton ball, an alcohol swab, and a bandage, placing them near the tray. I find it is easiest if I also unwrap the swab and the bandage so I don't have to fumble with the packaging during the process.

Next, choose the site for the shot. Since these are subcutaneous shots, it helps to pick an area where there is a little bit of fat under the surface. The most common sites for shots are in the abdomen and the tops of the thighs. These sites should be rotated from dose to dose. One easy way to remember this is to place a bright sticker on your calendar on the day when the shot is to be given. Use a different corner of the calendar square to indicate where the shot is to be given (upper right corner for right side of the abdomen, lower left side for the left thigh, etc.). Don't pick a site that is too close to a mole, a scar, a stretch mark, or an area where a vein is clearly visible below the surface. For the abdomen, pick a site that is at least two to three inches away from the belly button, as that is a very sensitive area.

Once you have gathered the equipment and chosen the site, it is time to get ready. Wash your hands thoroughly with soap and hot water, counting slowly to 20 while lathering up and rinsing. Dry your hands using paper towels. Some people choose to stand during the shot but I am not one of them. In fact, when I first started doing this, I was so sure that I would faint from the needle that I sat on the ground, figuring I would have a shorter distance to fall. Find a comfortable position. Using the alcohol swab, clean an area of the skin about four inches by four inches. Do not blow on the skin to dry it, as doing so potentially introduces more bacteria to the site. While the patch is drying, uncap the needle, placing the cap nearby. Turn the needle so that it points to the ceiling. Gently pressing the plunger, squeezing the air from the needle. If a small amount of medicine escapes, that's okay. Set the needle back on the tray or hold it in your dominant hand, almost the way you would hold a pencil or a dart. In your nondominant hand, gather the skin in a pinch so that about an inch-wide swath of skin arises.

At about a 45-degree angle to the skin, jab the needle quickly into the pinched skin until the needle sinks in and hits the hilt. Using the thumb of your dominant hand, draw the needle back just a little bit. If blood appears, it means that you have hit a blood vessel. If this happens, withdraw the needle, toss it into your sharps container, and start again with a new needle. Otherwise, press down on the needle, slowly releasing the medication. I count very slowly to 30 to make sure I take my time. If it starts to hurt during this time, breathe in through your nose and out through your mouth or otherwise distract yourself until the feeling passes, making sure to continue pressing slowly on the plunger. When the plunger hits the bottom, withdraw the needle and place it on the tray. Grab the cotton ball and hold it on the shot site but don't rub the site. Put a bandage on the site. If the site is bleeding, apply the bandage on top of the cotton ball.

Be sure to recap the needle as best you can and place it in a sharps container, which your doctor can provide. Dispose of the cotton ball in the toilet and throw the remaining wrappers and the used alcohol wipe in the trash.

See? That wasn't so bad, was it?

one trip a month. Then write the information on a calendar with the phone number and prescription numbers. I employ a technique that vets all over America use to remind dog owners to give monthly heart worm medication, by placing a bright sticker on the family calendar; each time I walk by the calendar, I am reminded to call in the prescription. Online pharmacies are particularly helpful in this regard as they send regular e-mail messages reminding their users to reorder medication ahead of time.

But if you still aren't able to go it alone, there are a number of different products to help you remember your medication, some very costly and others free. Only you will be able to determine what is right for you.

Finding the product

Pill boxes—Perhaps the most common way to remember to take your medication is the use of these plastic gadgets that are available in most pharmacies for under ten dollars. The best ones for home use tend to be the ones that you fill once a week and contain sections for morning, afternoon, evening, and bedtime dosages. With this device, you are easily able to see when you will be getting close to refill times, making last minute pharmacy runs less likely.

Lisa, who takes about twenty-seven pills a day for her CD, finds this to be an ideal solution. "I also write out a schedule and check off the meds as I take them because I am really bad at remembering some days," she said.

If you plan to be away from your house during the day for work or other appointments, take the medication with you in a portable pillbox kept in a pocket. If you keep your medication in your purse or briefcase, it is harder to remember since it is both out of sight and out of mind; with the pillbox in your pocket, you are likely to feel it and thus remember to take the contents of the box.

Alarm reminders—There are a number of products on the market to remind you to take your medication equipped with an alarm. Programmable wristwatches that chirp at pill time and flash the name of the medication, devices that attach to the bottom of pill bottles and sound an alarm when a dose is due, downloadable programs for personal computers that beep during certain points in the day, and an e-mail and beeper service that sends multiple daily reminders for medication are just some of the different alarm options available on the market. These services are generally priced anywhere from thirty dollars to one hundred dollars and are available in some pharmacies and through online shops.

Although these gadgets are great reminder tools, one obvious problem arises when the technology designed to remind us is not close at hand. The beeping pill containers, for example, could be blaring away while we run to the grocery store or the watches may be forgotten, left on the bedside table all day chirping an endless reminder that is not heard.

Dispensing machines—The most expensive option in the medication compliance market, these machines sound an alarm and discharge a dose of medication at specific times daily. Usually, these rest on a counter and are powered by electricity or batteries. You fill them up weekly and program the timers to dispense the medication at certain times. Then, every time you are expected to take a dose, the machine coughs up the medication into an adjoining tray. Some of these machines afford a wide variety of options and are incredibly complex, allowing the user to download information on compliance and send it through e-mail to a doctor, if need be.

Aside from the price of these wonders that range from one hundred dollars to nine hundred dollars, one drawback is that they aren't easily portable. Unless you are planning to be around the machine all day, you will likely miss a dose. Another is that they are somewhat complicated to program so if you haven't set the time on your DVD player, you may have difficulty with these devices.

IN A SENTENCE:

> *Utilizing a strategy or product can help ensure medication compliance.*

learning

Vitamins, Herbs, and Other Essential Nutrients

YOU ARE what you eat, the saying goes. While that may be true in many people, you likely have learned by this point that it can't necessarily be said of people with IBD. Some days, we don't eat. Other days, we do but it goes through us so fast that it is never absorbed.

Because malnutrition and malabsorption often accompany IBD, supplementation with vitamins, minerals, and other essential nutrients might be more than beneficial—it may be necessary. Slower functioning muscles, dizziness, irregular heartbeats, even death can result from the inability to digest and absorb a number of nutrients. Other vitamins and minerals may be needed in greater amounts to offset losses occurring because of the disease process. While none of these will cure the disease, they can help to ease symptoms, bolster nutritional status, and correct deficiencies.

Beyond those nutrients, alternative supplements in the form of herbal preparations may also help ease symptoms. While your doctor probably won't spout information on these different natural elements, they have become staples in natural medicine throughout the ages for easing intestinal discomfort.

A huge note of caution is important before we get to the list below. Prior to even purchasing any of these supplements or altering your diet to incorporate more of them, you absolutely must discuss it with your doctor. I can't emphasize that enough.

The vitamins, minerals and other nutrients

Folic acid is a synthesized form of folate, a water-soluble B vitamin. It acts to produce and repair DNA and RNA and helps to produce and maintain both red and white cells. Folic acid is especially important during pregnancy, as a deficiency of it has been linked to neural tube deformities in newborns.

There are a lot of theories as to why folic acid is in lower levels in the blood of IBD patients. Perhaps the rapid turnover of cells at the inflammation site requires more folic acid. Maybe folic acid in CD patients with small bowel involvement isn't absorbed because of inflammation. Could it be that a loss of appetite leads to less folate consumption? No one is really sure. What we do know is that low folic acid levels can lead to anemia, a common problem for people with IBD, and that people with diets low in folic acid had higher occurrence rates of colon cancers in some studies.

Folic acid supplements can be swallowed or injected. In the diet, the recommended amount of folic acid is 400 micrograms, a relatively attainable target. Some foods that are relatively high in folic acid include cereals, breads and other manufactured products that are fortified with folic acid, orange juice, asparagus, broccoli, beef and chicken liver, eggs, avocados, cantaloupe, and bananas.

Vitamin B_{12} is necessary in the body as it aids in the preservation of normal red blood cells and nerves and aids in the creation of DNA, the building block of cells. It cleaves to protein found in food but that bond is severed in the stomach and B_{12} is absorbed in the ileum.

The body has a ready store of B_{12}; however, in people with CD in the ileum or those who have ileal resections, B_{12} deficiency can occur over time. This deficiency can result in an increase of difficulty with memory, gas, constipation, confusion, weakness, fatigue, and a sore mouth. It may also manifest itself as anemia.

Only a tiny amount of B_{12} is needed in the diet each day to reach the recommended levels of 2.4 micrograms and is easily reached in a well-balanced diet. Vegans, individuals who consume only plant products, may have a harder time achieving the goal as the vitamin B_{12} is found in animal products such as eggs, beef, chicken, and fish; it is now also available in some fortified grain products such as bread and cereal. For those individuals who are still unable to absorb the vitamin through normal digestion, a nasal spray containing the vitamin or intramuscular injections are also available and should be taken regularly.

Vitamin E is primarily a fat-soluble vitamin, the main job of which is to protect cells from the natural products of metabolization called antioxidants. These free radicals are a factor in the aging process and may contribute to the formation of certain cancers.

While the recommended amount of the vitamin in the daily diet is easily obtained through the well-balanced diet for the vast majority of both healthy and ill individuals, some people with CD who have suffered small bowel loss through resection or disease activity may suffer a deficiency.

Interestingly, a small number of studies have been done regarding vitamin E in IBD. One small study found a benefit in pairing omega-3 fatty acids with vitamin E and theorized that the combination may be of use in the treatment of CD. Further, larger-scale studies are needed and may be conducted in the near future.

Vitamin E is found in foods like leafy green vegetables and vegetable oils such as safflower oil or corn oil. The amount recommended for the daily diet is 22 international units (IU). Supplements, also used by many with heart disease as it helps to protect LDL cholesterol from oxidation, are usually available in 400 IU doses, a small, elipitical, translucent yellow pill.

Two notes: First, if you are choosing a supplement, you may want one with alpha-tocopheryl, as this is the most potent form of vitamin E. As always, check with your doctor first. Second, vitamin E can act as an anticoagulant, meaning it inhibits clot formation. If you are taking vitamin E supplements, be sure to let your doctors know before any procedure or surgery.

Magnesium is a mineral for which every cell in the body has a use. In particular, it helps to strengthen bones and coordinates muscle and nerve functions. Magnesium comes into the body in higher quantities in leafy green vegetables, seeds, and nuts and leaves the body through urine, diarrhea, and **steatorrhea.**

And for a normal, healthy individual with a well-balanced diet, most likely magnesium is not a huge concern. But in the case of IBD, patients tend to have more diarrhea and steatorrhea than the general population. Issues of malabsorption may arise in the inflamed intestines and individuals with strictures or active disease who may avoid foods that are rich in magnesium. Also, the use of the diuretic Lasix for swollen joints can lead to a decrease in magnesium. Signs of magnesium deficiency include muscle cramps, numbness, tingling, coronary spasms, and confusion.

Currently, the amount of magnesium in the daily diet should be about 410 mgs for men and 320 mgs for women. Foods that may work a little better in individuals with CD or UC include bananas, baked potatoes without the skin, steamed broccoli florets, peanut butter, hummus, tahini, and avocados.

Potassium is another one of those minerals that is excreted in higher amounts in people with vomiting, chronic diarrhea, or steatorrhea. It also is found in high amounts in milk and certain raw fruits and vegetables, things not tolerated in some IBD patients.

Technically an electrolyte, potassium is necessary in electrical and cellular functions in the body, for building muscles, metabolizing carbohydrates, and synthesizing proteins. Normally, people take in anywhere from two to six grams in a balanced diet. Malabsorption of potassium in IBD can happen when the time the food takes to travel from the mouth to the anus is fast, leaving the potassium little chance to be absorbed.

Having a low level of potassium can be relatively hellish since a person can faint or succumb entirely due to a cardiac arrhythmia. Other potential symptoms include depression, weak muscles and bones, slow reflexes and dry skin. Painful charley horses that tend to occur at night may also be a signal that potassium is flagging.

Although they come in different shapes and sizes, potassium pills are at times large and somewhat difficult to swallow. Luckily, potassium is in a lot of foods that people with certain dietary restrictions due to IBD can still eat. Salmon, cod, sardines, baked potatoes, bananas, mushrooms, broccoli, and citrus juice all provide potassium in the diet in high amounts.

Iron is a highly essential mineral that is used throughout the body in the conduction and use of oxygen. It is found in the red blood cells and stored in the liver and in tissues in various areas. Thus, it is not a surprise to learn that iron deficiency can lead to weakness, fatigue, lessened cognitive function, and difficulty maintaining body temperature, since all of these functions require proper cellular function and oxygen supply.

The amount of iron that is recommended in the daily diet ranges by age and sex, from 8 to 18 mg. Women require more due to blood losses during monthly menstruation while men require less. Most people are able to achieve the recommended amounts through the consumption of animal products like shellfish, fish, red meat, white meat, and eggs, less so through certain grains, beans, and legumes.

In IBD, supplementation has long been the treatment for patients with anemia due to bleeding, a rather frequent occurrence given the nature of the diseases. In this case, some patients complain of constipation and nausea, feelings that can be abated if the supplement is taken with food. Also, it is important to know that iron absorption can interfere with calcium absorption so the two should be taken in doses separated by a few hours.

Calcium is another essential mineral, though owing more to the building of strong bones and teeth. The most common mineral found in the body, calcium also helps to transmit nerve responses, maintain a healthy heartbeat, coagulate blood, sustain muscle function, and stimulate hormone secretion and enzyme release. Calcium deficiency can lead to lower bone density that is linked to osteoporosis and the interruption of any of the previously mentioned functions.

In IBD, calcium is important for a few of reasons. It is not as readily absorbed in the diseased ileums of individuals with CD. Calcium helps to replace lost bone mass when steroids are being used and can help to reduce diarrhea due to fat malabsorption as it binds with the bile acids, making stools bulkier. Calcium-containing foods are primarily dairy foods, substances many people with IBD avoid due to real or perceived lactose intolerance. Major recent studies have found that calcium has been shown to reduce the occurrence of colon cancer.

There are a number of calcium supplements on the market and most contain vitamin D, a vitamin necessary for absorption of the mineral; Tums, the over the counter antacid preparation, also contains calcium and comes in pleasant flavors. Within the dairy group, hard cheeses and yogurt are sometimes more easily tolerated than milk itself. Also, it is found in shellfish, canned salmon, and sardines, and is an additive in certain enriched products such as cranberry and orange juices and cereal products. A wide variety of processed foods aimed at children are now enriched with the mineral as well.

Omega-3 polyunsaturated fatty acids have garnered the attention of the IBD community in the past several years. The interest sprouted not long ago when researchers, curious as to why certain cultures such as the Inuit tribes and other indigenous northern dwelling people had almost no IBD incidence, began to study the environmental and dietary factors that might play into this occurrence rate. They zeroed in on their disproportionately higher consumption of cold-water fish such as salmon and mackerel to their counterparts in North American regions where IBD incidence was markedly higher and consumption of these fish lower. The fish, it turned out, had high levels of a substance known as omega-3 fatty acids. Therefore, the researchers theorized, it stood to reason that by increasing the amount of this substance in the diets of IBD patients, perhaps a change could be made in their conditions. They felt that the fatty acids, offered in numerous giant capsules swallowed several times daily, offered a variety of mitigating effects on cellular activity in the inflammation process.

Since that time, several studies of various sizes, with various controls and methods have appeared on the subject, some with CD only, some with UC only, some with both, some in animal models, and some in humans. The results have been decidedly mixed. In some studies, a benefit for prolonging remission in IBD patients was found. However, human patients in the studies complained of a fishy odor that seemed to seep from their pores and arose in their breath. Special capsules that are coated to release the substance beyond the stomach seemed to help a little bit.

Omega-3 fatty acids have been studied for use in a number of diseases and are known to reduce the amounts of strokes and heart attacks in some individuals, reduce arthritis pain and ease the highs and lows of bipolar disorders. Certain foods that contain these include flaxseed and fish such as cod, salmon, mackerel, tuna, herring, and halibut.

Probiotics, prebiotics, and synbiotics

Probiotics are the use of two organisms that enhance and sustain each other's life; in current medicine, it commonly refers to the introduction of bacteria in the body to normalize function. Probiotics don't really fall into vitamins, herbs, or other essential nutrients, but they are very worthy of note as an additive to the diet, especially in light of various recent small studies. These studies have found that the addition of certain bacteria ingested in capsules have relieved diarrhea symptoms in various IBD patients.

The colon is the home of over four hundred different bacteria organisms, all living in a balance and serving a function in digestion. When the balance is disrupted due to disease activity or the use of antibiotics, diarrhea can result. The use of probiotics usually involves the reintroduction of certain bacteria such as lactobacillus GG, acidophilus, and bifidobacterium.

Doctors are beginning to suggest the use of probiotics more as an alternative, supplemental treatment of IBD, particularly in treating pouchitis. A recent study indicated that a certain formulation of probiotics, known as VSL#3, was helpful in controlling that condition. Another study is currently evaluating VSL#3 and a placebo in maintaining remission in CD. Still, there have yet to be large studies confirming the benefits of these supplements, and the controversy surrounding them continues.

While probiotics actually deliver more good bacteria to the colon, prebiotics act as food and energy sources for the beneficial bacteria there. The prebiotics are swallowed in pill form and go undigested until they hit the colon. If there are few studies regarding the beneficial effects of probiotics in IBD, there are far fewer regarding the use of prebiotics. In fact, of dozens of IBD studies now being conducted in the United States, only one is taking place currently to look at the potential dietary benefits of fructoogliosaccharides, a form of prebiotic. The results of that study are not expected until 2009.

Finally, synbiotics are combinations of probiotics and prebiotics, a sort of bacterial all-in-one package for the colon. These, too, are just beginning to be studied; a double-blind, placebo-controlled study in Scotland is looking into the potential beneficial effects of a synbiotic containing the prebiotic inulin and the probiotic bifidobacteria. The results of that study are expected in 2008.

Herbs

I've purposely saved herbal treatments for last, in part because the scientific community is just beginning to examine the potential benefits in the use of certain herbs for the relief of symptoms. In 1991, Congress passed legislation establishing within the National Institutes of Health an Office of Alternative Medicine, now the National Center for Complementary and Alternative Medicine, to examine the treatments using scientifically acceptable methods.

However, tribal medicine men and ancient midwives have been prescribing certain herbs for the relief of everything from pregnancy related nausea to digestive upset. You should check with your doctor about using some of these items prior even to purchasing these in your local health food store. You may also want to work with an herbalist to assure the proper usage and to learn of possible interactions between herbs and traditional medicines.

Peppermint, chamomile, and fennel seed tea—These teas have been used since ancient times to relax the intestinal muscles, soothe spasms and ease colic. Peppermint can also be swallowed in enteric-coated capsules or its leaves can be plucked directly from the living plant and chewed. People with reflux may find that these teas or remedies exacerbate that condition as they help to relax the lower esophageal sphincter, worsening the flow of acid into the esophagus.

Ginger root, coriander seed, and cilantro—For millennia, women have nibbled on ginger root, coriander seeds, and cilantro to relieve nausea associated with pregnancy. The good news is that these may also relieve nausea associated with other conditions as well.

Black cohosh tea and evening primrose oil—In at least one study, women with IBD report greater premenstrual symptoms and pain associated with their menstrual cycle. However, most PMS-pain products contain ibuprofen that can further exacerbate IBD symptoms. For relief, some women turn to evening primrose oil in capsule form or brew themselves cups of black cohosh tea. Neither of these is associated with negative GI symptoms.

Dong Quai—Used as a tincture or in pill form, this Chinese herb acts as an antispasmodic by relaxing the smooth muscle. It is also used to reduce PMS and menopausal symptoms.

Slippery elm bark—Used as survival food by the early American settlers, this bark can be made into a gruel, is found in capsules and in freeze dried formula. It is known as mucilage, a sticky, slippery substance that coats the intestines and helps to soothe inflammation.

IN A SENTENCE:

> *A well balanced diet usually supplies adequate essential nutrients in most people, but IBD patients may find they need supplements to correct deficiencies.*

living

Seeking
Alternative Therapy

AMERICANS LOVE alternative therapies. This is not only an observation but also a statement of fact. In the past few years, as yoga studios blossomed in strip malls across America and wheat grass concoctions became common at juice bars, we learned that about 40 percent of Americans put their hopes in more natural means of health by swallowing $1.7 billion in dietary supplements, according to the National Health and Nutrition Examination Survey. In 1997 alone, 42 percent of Americans spent $27 billion on complementary and alternative therapies. That figure reflected a 9 percent increase in the number of Americans seeking such treatment since 1990.

And the government, sensing this was more of a change in medicine than a fad, in 1991 opened an office through the National Institutes of Health to study—and ultimately prove or debunk—certain alternative remedies. The National Center for Complementary and Alternative Medicine monitors research that applies the current Western gold standards of double-blind, randomized, placebo-controlled, multicenter studies, to the more Eastern practices of acupuncture and herbal remedies such as St. John's wort.

Doctors are also changing the way they practice medicine. One study found that 60 percent prescribe anything from vitamin and herbal supplements to tai chi classes. Another noted that about three-quarters of the nation's medical schools teach students about available complementary and alternative medicine.

But just because everyone seems to be doing it or because the government has studied certain therapies doesn't mean you should go out and give it a go on your own. Your doctor is essentially the coordinator of your care and as such needs to know exactly what you are taking or what you are doing, if for no other reason than to guard against potentially dangerous interactions between some herbs and some medications. For example, St. John's wort and cyclosporine have an interaction that makes the immune suppressant less effective, something your doctor could warn you about. Also, your doctor may be able to advise you on the proper amount of a certain supplement to take or to supply you with research on the effectiveness of acupuncture, for example. You may also be surprised to obtain a referral from your doctor regarding certain alternative practitioners.

Finding a practitioner

If you are looking to try an alternative approach to treatment and have spoken with your doctor about it, you may first want to learn as much as you can about the particular therapy you are investigating before going into the closest practitioner's office. There are numerous books available on everything from acupuncture to chiropractic methods, from homeopathy to naturopathy, and thousands of Web sites dedicated to each on the Internet.

Ask your doctor, friends, and relatives for references for individual practitioners. Ask them what their experience has been, both good and bad. Scour the national organizations related to the field for local practitioners in your area, but beware that many of these organizations do not operate in the same manner as the national medical boards and organizations for doctors. While some offer continuing education and uphold strict standards, others require little more than an annual fee to be listed. It will pay in the long run to find out what their standards are.

Find out where the practitioner is located, how much treatment costs, and whether or not insurance will cover the trip. Some insurance will cover such things as a visit to the chiropractor for an adjustment or a few visits to the acupuncturist. However, most insurance policies either have restrictions on the amount of coverage or don't cover the practice at all.

Checking out the individual's credentials is harder than it is with physicians. Some states have regulatory boards or agencies for specific fields of alternative medicine such as naturopathy, homeopathy, or chiropractic medicine, and require licensing; these agencies should be able to provide you with information on the individual's education and training, as well as any disciplinary actions taken against them. Many states do not have very extensive bureaucracy to monitor the individuals. In this case, a trip to your local district court may yield information about the individual's background, particularly if a lawsuit has been filed against them; you may want to inquire about the individual through the local chamber of commerce as well, as they usually share information or complaints about the practitioner.

Before agreeing to the treatment, make a time to talk to the practitioner about what he or she will be doing for or to you. Discuss his or her attitudes about continuing more traditional medical treatment and how he or she will work with your doctor. A huge warning sign you may encounter is if an alternative medical practitioner advises you to discontinue all traditional therapy or says she or she can cure you. Run, don't walk, out of that office if this occurs. Take a look at the facility: the floor, the walls, the cabinets, the bathrooms. If these are not clean and in good shape, leave.

Here are some other questions you may want to ask:

1. What kind of education and training did you receive in your profession?
2. Do you have any certification or formal license to practice?
3. How long have you been practicing this alternative therapy?
4. Do all patients respond positively? (another flag question)
5. How many patients do you see in a day?
6. Do you work with anyone else in case you are not available?
7. How long do you spend with each patient?
8. How many treatments are typically required in a situation such as mine?
9. What exactly will you be doing with me?
10. How do you clean any instruments you use?
11. Will there be anything I am required to do at home?
12. Are there any side effects to this treatment?

13. Do you have any scientific information to back up the efficacy and safety of this process?

This last question is also a potential flag. Some therapies can be backed up with scientific studies that show their benefit or safety; others can't. If your practitioner can't point to studies, it may be because they don't exist. This isn't necessarily a bad thing, since many alternative treatments haven't been documented in this fashion. Still, you need to see what is out there and judge whether or not you are comfortable with its evidence or lack thereof.

Finding treatments and "cures" on the Web

There are literally thousands of pages on the Internet devoted to products that claim to treat or cure IBD through the use of special manipulation techniques or supplements. Simple herbal treatments including aloe concoctions and more complex chemical formulations so difficult to pronounce that they go by initials only are offered with a few mouse clicks.

While some vitamins and herbs can help with symptoms and are offered at bargain prices through online stores, some of the stuff offered has no benefit whatsoever. Instead of a "cure" for your disease, you could be relieved of nothing but your hard earned dollars.

As the leader of an Internet bulletin board for Crohn's patients, I am often asked what I think about these miracle products. Here are some key things to take note of when wondering whether an item would be beneficial to your health:

1. A site that touts the health benefits of a product without real studies to back it up. One particular site about which a friend asked my opinion featured bovine colostrum, the first milk a mother cow would produce to feed to a calf. This site gave a lot of information about the product, including testimonials from users who claimed to be cured of symptoms. One particular link that supplied "proof" of the manufacturer's claims led to a story of a dog named Fluffy that was cured of a degenerative disc condition that was often found in his breed through drinking small amounts of the cow milk. Of the two dozen reference links, not one pointed to a credible study that could be accessed in its entirety.

2. A product that claims to relieve a variety of ailments. I am not talking three or four related conditions like CD, UC, and ulcerative proctitis. Rather, I refer to products that claim to provide relief or a cure for unrelated conditions from warts to muscular twitches to AIDS and everything in between. No elixir is magical enough to do it all.

3. A product that is available on "this site only." If "Mrs. X's Snake Oil" is truly good, well-tested, safe, and efficacious, it will likely be available in other areas. Same thing goes for those sites that say "supplies are limited."

4. If you can order the product directly from the Web site, don't buy it. Chances are the information that accompanies the material will offer nothing but glowing reviews. Gone will be the studies or other information that casts even a slightly negative light on the product.

If any question remains, print out a copy of the site and bring it to your doctor for discussion.

A *note on the danger of colonics*

Stars like Alicia Silverstone rave about it. Princess Diana was reported to steal away to a London clinic three times a week for it. It must be great, right?

"It" is colon hydrotherapy, also known as colonics or high enemas. Practitioners of these alternative therapies perform them by placing the recipient either on their backs or on their sides and inserting an enema tip four to five inches into the rectum. Varying amounts of tap water, coffee, or herbal potions are then released by pump or gravity into the colon. The substance then allegedly loosens from the colon wall fecal matter, some of which some practitioners say has been in the colon for years. The liquid and solid remains of the treatment are either emptied through the same tube or are expelled out during ensuing bowel movements. Some Web sites extolling the virtues of these treatments show these contents proudly displayed on sheets, the ground, aluminum pie plates, or in rubber gloved hands. Other sites sell equipment that looks more like a medieval torture device, complete with a large tank that when filled with water slowly empties into the waiting colon.

Offering no suitable scientific information to back up their claims, the practitioners of colon hydrotherapy say that they can cure everything from acne to body odor and of course all intestinal ailments through cleansing the colon of "toxins" that build up in it and release all sorts of dangerous materials into the blood. They say that the recipient of this therapy often will feel a "healing crisis" that follows the enema but not to be worried since the fever, chills, uncontrollable shaking, and faintness is just the result of the damage being slowly undone. After several of these treatments, the individual can move into more of a maintenance mode, having the procedure done four times a year.

Colon hydrotherapy is a drain on your bank account at best and life-threatening at worst. Practitioners with little knowledge of anatomy or physiology have been known to perforate the rectum, causing life-threatening gangrene. The therapies also cause a loss of electrolytes such as sodium, magnesium, and potassium, causing everything from cramping and chills to heart arrhythmias. Some use equipment over and over without putting it through the high-temperature process called autoclaving, potentially exposing recipients to a host of different infectious agents.

In the case of IBD, these procedures can be particularly damaging. The inflamed mucosa can be irritated by the enema process or contents, causing more bleeding. Individuals with strictures can experience pain and possibly perforation with the increased colon contents. Tender rectums can be punctured by the enema applicators.

This process is not to be confused with the lavage performed prior to a colonoscopy. The colon cleansing process for that procedure is used to remove normal bits of waste and effluent to allow for an easier time of viewing by the physician.

The colon does not need cleansing otherwise. It contains a balanced mini-ecosystem of about four hundred different kinds of bacteria that work together in the digestion and absorption process. When the bacteria die, they join the fecal matter in exiting the body. We depend on the bacteria and they depend on us. Food particles rarely stick around for more than a couple of days—not months or years as the colon hydrotherapy folks would have you believe.

IN A SENTENCE:

> *Before using an alternative therapy, consult your doctor, and use caution in selecting the practitioner.*

FIRST-MONTH MILESTONE

By the end of the first month, you have moved further in the quest for knowledge and understanding of the disease by:

○ LEARNING THAT THERE IS NO MEDICAL CURE FOR THE DISEASE BUT THERE IS AN ARSENAL OF PRESCRIPTION MEDICATIONS TO CONTROL SYMPTOMS AND SLOW OR HALT INFLAMMATION;

○ BEING INTRODUCED TO ADAPTABLE STRATEGIES FOR TAKING THE MEDICATION AND TO CONTROL ITS SIDE EFFECTS; AND

○ DISCOVERING THE POTENTIAL BENEFITS OF VITAMINS, HERBS, AND OTHER ALTERNATIVE TREATMENTS.

The Role of Nutrition

FOR THE most part, people with IBD are able to retain a good nutritional profile during most of their lives through the consumption of a balanced diet. Good portions of well-absorbed protein, fats, and carbohydrates, as well as micronutrients like vitamins and minerals, help to keep our bones and muscles strong, maintain healthy body weight, and avoid further injury through diseases and conditions related to malnutrition.

Many IBD patients can and do consume a full diet either in the presence or absence of disease activity or scar tissue. Dietary supplements can make up for any shortfall. Special diets may be needed to ease certain symptoms such as a low-fat diet for fat malabsorption or a clear liquid diet following surgery or in preparation for a colonoscopy.

As you may have discovered on your own up to this point, IBD patients have a hard time maintaining their weight as well as their nutritional status due to disease activity in the digestive tract. As discussed in Week 4, some vitamins and minerals are not as easily absorbed due to inflammation and scar tissue.

Weight loss is of particular concern as it generally reflects serious disease activity. Malnourishment sets a terrible cycle in motion that lessens the body's ability to recover without adequate nutrition. Disease activity can worsen, making nutrition a nearly impossible goal. For these people, nutrition intervention is important.

The malnutrition can occur for several reasons. Anorexia happens when the patient sees that his or her digestive symptoms are related to the consumption of food. By eliminating or reducing the amount that is brought into the body, it will hence reduce the amount exiting the body, the thought goes. Pain and nausea are constant companions to the patient and the physical prompt makes it easier to avoid eating. But by reducing food intake, the patient is also reducing the body's chances of being well-nourished. Without the proper amounts of protein, carbohydrates, fats, vitamins, and minerals, the body burns protein found in muscles and bones, weakening both. For some, the issue is more **cachexia** than anorexia. In this instance, individuals eat normal amounts of food but not enough to meet the body's increased needs that relate to greater metabolic action due to fever and to the inflammatory process.

Still more individuals with IBD—nearly all CD as opposed to UC patients—suffer from some level of malabsorption related to disease activity. These people are not able to absorb nutrients due to inflammation or scar tissue impeding the natural digestive process. Sometimes, an underlying motility disorder speeds up the pace at which food normally travels through the small bowel, leaving little opportunity for normal absorption. And a small number of CD patients suffer from **short bowel syndrome,** a condition caused by surgical removal of large portions of the small bowel. With less gut to absorb nutrients, the patients can slowly starve to death without intervention.

Aiding the malnourished patient

To rectify a malnourished patient's nutritional status, doctors often first encourage good nutrition, especially to those who may simply avoid eating due to anorexia. They may gently suggest to the patient alternatives to eating, such as consuming liquid nutrients in the form of defined formula diets. Ready-made drinks such as Boost, Ensure, Sustacal, and Isocal are widely available in pharmacies and grocery stores, are easily absorbed in the small intestine, and provide complete nutrition. They are palatable, come in a handful of flavors, and are best served cold; some manufacturers have come out with a line of such nutritionally complete food items as relatively tasty nutrition bars and puddings. These products supply up to 1,200 nutrition-rich calories per serving, come in milk-free formulas, and are easily incorporated into the daily diet.

But when eating is impossible due to severe disease activity, because the defined formula diets are unpalatable, or when the bowel is significantly shortened by surgery, a doctor may prescribe an **elemental diet.** Elemental diets are nutritionally complete, like their defined formula counterparts, but they are readily absorbed, requiring very little activity on the part of the stomach or intestines. Depending on the situation, some people on elemental diets can still eat varying amounts of normal food during this treatment. However, prescription formulas can have an awful metallic taste and very little can be done to change this. Aside from this, people often have to swallow the somewhat expensive concoctions several times daily. To avoid the taste, some people insert the elemental concoctions into the stomach via a nasogastric tube. Others have a PEG (percutaneous endoscopic gastrostomy) tube inserted into the stomach to allow the formula to pass through to the stomach, bypassing the mouth or nasogastric tube altogether.

Total parenteral nutrition (TPN) is generally reserved for individuals who suffer from short bowel and those for whom bowel rest is prescribed. The concept of using TPN as therapy is controversial but it works well to sustain nutrition in the aforementioned individuals. In this form of feeding, a catheter is placed either in a vein in the arm or in the upper chest. Through the catheter, a solution of nutrients is dripped into the body and can include minerals such as potassium, magnesium, and sodium, as well as vitamins, carbohydrates, and fats. Although TPN is started in the hospital, it can be continued at home, with the individual hooking up bags of nutrients to the line and infusing them throughout the night. Night drips allow the individual more freedom during the day.

TPN is not without its risks. Continuous feedings can lead to liver damage in a small number of patients while others may experience blood-borne bacterial infections leading to sepsis. Thrombosis, the clotting within the

CROHN'S DISEASE AND ULCERATIVE COLITIS

major vein, is another serious consequence some patients face while on TPN. It is also not without cost. The average annual cost of TPN exceeds $150,000, some of which may not be covered by insurance.

IN A SENTENCE:

> *Nutritional therapies can help maintain health in individuals who avoid eating or can't absorb proper amounts of nutrients.*

living

What Can I Eat?
What Should I Avoid?

WHEN ASKED these questions, many doctors offer a pat answer: Eat what you want unless it bothers you. They may add a few restrictions like low-fiber or low-fat or iron rich but beyond that, you are on your own.

Part of the blame for this common shrugging of the shoulders falls on the medical schools for not providing nearly enough education to the doctors on the subject of diet and nutrition. In textbooks on GI diseases, huge portions are dedicated to the pathological implications of the disease, the effects of the various medications, and the spectacular array of surgical options, but one thin chapter is devoted to diet. IBD textbooks are no different. Within the one chapter on diet, much information will be given on enteral feeding, the proper mixture and additives to TPN, and the effects of short bowel syndrome, but nothing is offered on giving nutrition advice or suggestions to patients who fall short of those dire circumstances.

Even when doctors do hand out diet information sheets, they give very little information outside which foods are to be embraced and which are to be shunned. There are usually no recipes or suggestions for eating away from home, and no information on jazzing up a so-called bland diet or making a liquid diet more than chicken or beef broth.

And yet, many doctors say that one of the first questions out of a patient's mouth has to do with their diet. While no food has been found to be the cause of CD or UC, certain foods most assuredly exacerbate symptoms in some individuals.

Fat

Fat is one of those things that we need for living. Although it doesn't contain vital nutrients, it does provide twice as many calories as protein and carbohydrates, and we burn those extra calories for energy. Fat is also needed for the absorption of vitamins A, D, E, and K. But in people with IBD, fat can come as a catch-22—we need it but it can make our lives miserable.

For one, fat is a powerful stimulant to the GI tract. Remember that bag of fries you inhaled and then chased with a greasy burger? Now think back to how quickly you felt the effects of it and how fast you had to dash to the bathroom. After swallowing a greasy meal, the peristaltic activity in just about everyone is increased. For those with a propensity for diarrhea, that activity is not welcome. Add to this the fact that some individuals with IBD have the underlying motility disorder IBS, and you have a recipe for both increased bathroom time and toilet paper consumption.

Secondly, people with CD involving ileal disease or resections often do not absorb fats as well as individuals without ileal disease. The type of diarrhea that results from this lack of absorption is called steatorrhea and is characterized by bad smelling, poorly formed feces that float in the toilet. While this condition can come and go with disease activity, some people struggle with this forever after bowel resections due to the decrease in bile acid that is absorbed and reused by the intestines. For these individuals, the drug Questran can help to bind the stools.

In either case, reducing dietary fat can reduce diarrhea activity in many individuals with IBD. Avoiding fast food is one step in the process. Anything fried—from seemingly innocuous traditional potato chips to the more blatantly obvious fried chicken—may cause an increase in diarrhea.

Looking for other sources of fat such as in egg yolks, mayonnaise, cooking oil, certain dairy products and desserts, butter, and margarine will help you to identify fat sources and develop a strategy for avoiding them.

Caffeine

My husband always believed that he couldn't start the day without a cup of strong coffee and a sports section. But when the local newspapers went on strike, he found that he could still have a bowel movement without the aid of football stories. However, when we ran out of coffee and neither of us could get to the store for a few days, he became anxious. Aside from the caffeine-withdrawal headache, he didn't have the extra push to help him evacuate his bowels in the morning.

My husband is not alone. Many people rely on the bowel-activating stimulus caffeine provides in order to get things moving. The problem arises in people with active IBD who need no extra stimulation for their bowels.

Colas, coffee, certain teas, and chocolate all contain varying amounts of caffeine. Herbal tea offers a good solution particularly if it contains peppermint, fennel, or chamomile, all known for their soothing effects on the GI tract.

Alcohol

There is a lot to be said in the negative regarding alcohol. For one, it inhibits folic acid absorption. Alcohol is an irritant to the GI tract, and using alcohol is one of the major contributing factors to pancreatitis. It is the second greatest factor in the development of cirrhosis of the liver (viral hepatitis C holds first place). It is filled with empty calories that often take the place of valuable nutrients.

In IBD, it can lead to an increase in diarrhea in some individuals, especially if the alcohol is wine that contains sulfites and the individual is sensitive to sulfites. Of course, everyone is different and some people will feel no ill effect. The amount ingested and whether it accompanies food also are factors in the degree of affect. However, alcohol also should not be ingested when on immunosuppressants such as 6-MP or while taking Flagyl.

Dairy products

An excellent provider of calcium, dairy foods in general are also a source of lactose, a milk sugar that is broken down with the help of the enzyme lactase. If you are lacking this enzyme (produced in the small intestine), bacteria in the colon feed on the undigested sugar and produce hydrogen, which leads to diarrhea and to the build up of gas in the intestines. Many people with UC tend to have this condition whether they have disease activity or not, and other IBD patients develop symptoms of it with the presence of active disease.

To avoid the unpleasant physical effects of lactose intolerance, many IBD patients avoid milk and dairy products entirely. However, there are certain dairy products that they may be able to tolerate such as yogurt (Dannon or Breyers brands that are not highly processed) or small amounts of firm, aged cheeses. With the reduction of dairy products, some effort should be made to supplement the diet with vitamin D and calcium.

Carbonated beverages and other gas-producing foods and drinks

While it is true that we all pass gas, people with IBD may find the process of gas buildup in the intestines more painful than those with healthy intestines. It may also be more perplexing as it can accompany fecal incontinence in some.

For these reasons, it might be wise to dodge beverages such as pop or beer that contain carbonation, the gasses and fermentation of which can lead to uncomfortable bloating. Substituting herbal tea, lemonade, or other noncarbonated, noncaffeinated beverages might help. Gas-producing foods may also be avoided during disease activity if they cause a problem. Broccoli, certain beans, garlic, onions, leeks, cauliflower, and cabbage all are sulfur-producing vegetables, tending to produce more gas in the consumer. Exchanging these vegetables for other, less gaseous vegetables such as carrots might be an option for those struggling with gas.

Red meat

There is nothing like the taste of a hot, juicy roast beef sandwich on a cold winter day or a tender steak right off the grill during a summer picnic. But in people with UC, the consumption of red meat—in addition to eggs and certain milk products—may lead to the increase in the production of hydrogen sulfide in the colon, a circumstance that has a negative effect on the health of the colonic mucosa.

At least one study has shown that avoiding red meat leads to greatly lower hydrogen sulfide levels and other studies have documented a lessening of symptoms among individuals with active UC who avoided these foods.

Still, dropping beef from the diet is a hard thing to do in a red meat-loving nation. There is life after red meat, I promise you. Beyond tuna and salmon, more and different varieties of fish are available in most grocery stores; often in restaurants it is served with steamed vegetables and a rice dish, a perfect option. Chicken is versatile as are soy products such as tofu. Textured vegetable protein (TVP) has made it to the store shelves, seasoned for use as a substitute for meat in chili or in bolognese sauces.

Artificial fats and sweeteners

On the surface, these items would seem to be the perfect solution to reducing dietary fat and excess sugar in the diet as these relatively new products seek to avoid the consequences of consuming too much of these potentially diet-busting substances.

But individuals with IBD may want to avoid them, since many of these products carry warnings that they also carry a risk of diarrhea. Sorbitol is one example. Found in many sugarless chewing gums, cookies, and numerous other sweets, this synthetic sugar substitute is a known cause of diarrhea in healthy people. Olestra is another, as the fake fat coats the intestinal walls and causes diarrhea, as well as a host of other painful and embarrassing digestive symptoms, even in otherwise healthy individuals.

Instead of incorporating these items in the diet, look for ways to reduce fats and sugars through other means. Eat baked potato chips instead of olestra chips or fried ones. Consume small amounts of sugar instead of large amounts or sugar substitutes.

Fructose

Many people consider fruit—right up there with vegetables—as an essential part of a healthy diet. And indeed, for most people, these delicious foods are not a problem to digest. Because the vast majority of the population can tolerate fruit, fructose, the sugar derived from fruit, is often added to foods to provide a kick of sweetness, including the ubiquitous high fructose corn syrup.

But for a relatively small percentage of the population, consuming fructose can send them to the bathroom with bloating, cramping, and diarrhea. That's because these individuals lack the enzyme to break down the sugar, thus allowing the colon bacteria to consume it and cause the digestive complaints as a result. This is not unlike lactose intolerance.

For individuals who feel that fructose might be a problem, studies have found that avoidance of the sugar helps relieve symptoms. A good selection of vegetables can make up for any nutritional differences. Also, checking for the sugar in manufactured foods can go a long way in preventing discomfort caused by fructose intolerance.

Fiber

Your doctor may have told you to add fiber to your diet to help gel your stools. Or maybe he or she told you to reduce fiber to avoid an obstruction at a stricture. You've probably heard that fiber is a laxative—and that is the last thing you need when you are already running to the bathroom a dozen times in a day. But likely no one told you how fiber works in the GI tract, how we get it, or that there are two kinds of fiber.

First, let's start with the two kinds of fiber: insoluble and soluble. Insoluble fiber is the kind that is often found in raw fruits and vegetables as well as in certain grains. This fiber, as the name implies, does not take on water in the gut but rather provides undigested bulk to the stool, a great plus for people who are suffering from constipation. Various leafy greens and brans contain insoluble fiber, as do the skins and seeds of just about all fruits and vegetables. Nuts, a great source of nutrients, unfortunately also contain insoluble fiber.

Soluble fiber is found in a variety of grain products as well as a few vegetables. Unlike its counterpart, soluble fiber takes on water, providing bulk
to the stools. One good test of this is by submerging foods in a glass of
water; if the food takes on water, it probably contains soluble fiber. Think
oatmeal, white bread, white rice, pasta, and potatoes, and you are thinking soluble fiber. Dried peas and beans both combine soluble fiber (they
absorb water when soaked in it) and insoluble fiber (the tiny, tough jackets that surround them).

Insoluble fiber does not easily pass through strictures in the intestine
and can contribute to an obstruction at the site of one. It can also irritate
an already inflamed gut. For these reasons, it is wise to avoid all whole nuts,
raw fruits, raw vegetables, their skins, and seeds during times when inflammation or scar tissue cause intestinal narrowing. The nutrients from these
foods are too important to forgo entirely, however. One way to reduce the
fiber is to break down the fiber matrix through steaming or baking the fruits
or vegetables until they are "fork tender," meaning they can be easily
squashed with the back of a fork. Nut flours or nut butters are easier to
digest as the matrix has been pulverized.

Increasing soluble fiber is a tasty and easy way to help wick up some of
the excess, unabsorbed fluid in the intestines. Incorporating more foods
containing soluble fiber or such products as Metamucil, Citrucel, or Fiber-
Con can help to provide a stabilizing agent to the watery intestinal contents, making stools more gel-like than liquid in nature. These foods also
tend to be easy to incorporate in the diet during a flareup when only bland,
soothing foods seem to be tolerated.

Surviving special diets

Low-fat, low-fiber, low-salt, clear liquid, soft foods, iron-rich, lactose
free. You name it, there seems to be some application of nearly every imaginable diet for people with IBD at some stage in their disease. For the most
part, these are temporary, lasting anywhere from a day for the colonoscopy
prep to a few weeks until bad symptoms subside or the medication can be
withdrawn.

Still, it is difficult to live with these special diets when everyone around
you is able to dig in to their regular, delicious meals without a care. Meals

at restaurants or family celebrations become torture as you are relegated to a narrow list of foods.

Low-fat diet

○ This diet helps with people who are unable to absorb fats or find that fatty foods lead to multiple bowel movements.

○ Learn to prepare your own dishes at home if you don't already. Although low-fat options abound in the market, plenty of prepared foods contain unhealthy amounts of fat. By fixing your own foods, you will have a greater control over fat content.

○ Use nonstick pans as they require little to no oil for cooking. For other pans, use Pam cooking spray lightly.

○ Learn safe substitutes for fat. For example, use two egg whites where a recipe calls for one whole egg, reduce the amount of oil in a recipe, substitute applesauce for oil where possible, buy textured vegetable protein (TVP) instead of meat for foods with sauce such as spaghetti, try hard cheese as opposed to soft cheeses that are higher in fat, and buy low fat versions of regular staples (salad dressing, mayonnaise, etc.).

○ Trade your high fat snacks for lower-fat versions.

○ Look for "heart-healthy" entrees in restaurants, as these are usually low in fat.

Low-fiber diet

○ This is usually prescribed for individuals who have stricturing disease.

○ Learn to prepare your own dishes at home if you don't already, but don't be afraid to include other prepared foods as some are naturally low in fiber.

○ Cook all raw fruits and vegetables that you cannot squash easily with a fork. Avocados, bananas, ripe mangos, and melons are fairly easy to squash because their fiber matrix is not as intense and can be eaten raw. However, fruits and vegetables such as apples, broccoli, and spinach should be steamed or baked until they are easily squashed with a fork.

○ Avoid items such as whole wheat bread or wild rice or any other food where the insoluble portion of fiber is clearly visible.

○ If nuts are required in a recipe, use a fine grinder, food processor, or food mill instead of rough chopping them.

○ Avoid tough, stringy meats. Ground meats such as ground sirloin are easier to digest.

○ Chew your food well and take your time when eating.

○ Ask your doctor about supplementing your diet with a multivitamin to cover any nutrients you may have to cook out of the fruits and vegetables you consume.

Low-salt diet

○ This diet may help reduce bloating associated with prednisone usage.

○ Read the ingredient listing and nutritional label for sodium content. You may be surprised by which products contain sodium.

○ Because more processed foods contain sodium, focus on preparing most of the food yourself.

○ Incorporate other powerfully flavored ingredients such as lemons, fresh herbs, garlic, shallots, and onions to boost the taste factor in meals without adding salt. Use salt-free spice mixes such as the Mrs. Dash line of spices to flavor meats and vegetables.

○ When eating out, avoid soups and sauces as many include salt as a chief ingredient.

○ When bloating does occur, look to natural diuretics like garlic, watermelon, asparagus, and licorice to reduce water gain.

Clear liquids and soft-foods diets

○ The clear liquid diets is usually prescribed in the case of a partial obstruction, following surgery, or in preparation for a colonoscopy; soft foods are usually the next step before resuming a full diet.

○ Notice that clear liquid and soft foods does not also say bland. That is because there is no reason these diets have to be totally bland. Choose foods such as lemon ice or pineapple Jell-O to liven up the day. Try herbal tea flavors you have never tried before.

○ Chicken and beef broth are a staple of these diets but they needn't be boring. Before adding the broth to a pan for heating, sauté crushed garlic cloves and diced onions or shallots in a tiny amount of oil until the onions become translucent. Then add the broth, straining the flavor additives out before serving. Other vegetables such as carrots and celery or herbs such as dill and basil also boost flavor and can be added to the soup pot for half an hour before being strained out.

○ When you are in the hospital and on these diets, you are at the mercy of the hospital kitchen. However, you can always bring your own tea bags and other clear or soft food items for a change of pace.

○ Soft foods such as oatmeal and eggs can be made more palatable with the additions of condiments, sweeteners, and spices like brown sugar, cinnamon, barbecue sauce, ketchup, soy sauce, or mustard.

Iron-rich diet

○ This diet is usually prescribed for individuals with anemia.

○ Cook your foods in cast iron pans, using Pam to ease food sticking and scorching.

○ Consume cereals that are fortified with iron.

○ Avoid taking your calcium supplement at the same time as the iron supplement, as absorption will be diminished. Take your supplement with orange juice, as it aids in absorption.

○ Avoid iron-rich foods that contain oxalic acids in abundance, as these can promote the development of kidney stones.

○ Try organ meats and red meats, as they are rich in iron. Wash the meal down with a glass of red wine.

Lactose-free diet

○ This diet is usually prescribed for individuals with lactose intolerance.

○ Learn to prepare your own dishes at home if you don't already. Although many dairy-free options abound in the market, plenty of prepared foods contain milk or milk products. By preparing your own foods, you will have a greater control over dairy content.

○ Read the label. Plenty of seemingly innocuous foods contain milk or milk products.

○ When shopping, look for lactose-free milk alternatives such as Lactaid, a milk product without lactose, or milk made from soy, almond, or rice milk. Try a few brands and even a few flavors within a brand until you find a match. Soy-based cheeses and other traditionally milk-based items can be quite nasty but some are also surprisingly good. A favorite of mine is the Tofutti brand ice cream sandwiches called Tofutti Cuties.

○ Look on the labels of food for kosher symbols without a "D" next to them or with the word "pareve" next to the label. Jewish dietary laws prohibit the mixing of milk with meat, and thus the D will appear on foods containing dairy, while pareve means that it has neither milk nor meat in it.

○ Try other plant-based sauces in place of milk-based sauces. Eat the marinara instead of the Alfredo; try salsa instead of French onion dip.

IN A SENTENCE:

> *While no foods are the cause of IBD, you may want to avoid certain foods and embrace others when trying to control diarrhea.*

learning

Non-Ostomy Surgical Options

THE EMPHASIS of treatment in IBD is generally to preserve the intestines through the use of medical treatment. Even in the direst of conditions, doctors at times will try to treat the patient first with medicine before resorting to surgery.

However, sometimes surgery is the only or best treatment available. And in most IBD patients, surgery will likely occur at least once in their lives. You may not have had one in the three months since you were diagnosed, but studies show that anywhere from 50 to 60 percent of Crohn's patients and about one-third of UC patients require at least one surgery in their lifetimes. Additionally, about 80 percent of those requiring one surgery must have a second surgery within twenty years of the first surgery.

The reasons for surgery are many and are dictated by the specific conditions relating to the individual. Some are life-threatening conditions that require emergency procedures while others are conditions that deteriorate slowly to the point where surgery is the only treatment option. Here are some of the more common reasons for surgery:

○ Medical treatment failure. Up to half of all patients on steroid therapy will not be able to achieve remission two years after starting the medication. Similarly, others are not responsive to other therapies such as the 5-ASA drugs or are unable to use immunomodulators.

○ Fulminant colitis and toxic megacolon. Many who suffer from these conditions must undergo emergency surgery.

○ Fistulas and abscesses. Remicade and antibiotics help to heal some of these formations in CD patients but others must undergo surgery to remove the diseased intestinal segment or drain the abscesses.

○ Strictures and obstructions. Inflammation can be the culprit in these instances and can be controlled by steroids, immune suppressors, and biologic medication. However, immovable and untreatable scar tissue can also cause these formations.

○ Perforation. An emergency condition, it must be corrected with immediate surgery, followed with antibiotic treatment.

○ Hemorrhage. Another emergency condition, this rare event is treated with surgery.

○ Colorectal cancer or risk of it. Common in UC and in Crohn's colitis, cancer usually calls for the removal of the colon.

○ Control of extraintestinal manifestations. Sometimes, conditions such as IBD-related eye conditions and arthritis will calm down only with the removal of the diseased segment of intestines.

For the most part, these surgeries are done in the traditional manner but an increasing number are being done with the use of laparoscopic technology. This technique involves an endoscopic-like device that enters the body cavity through a few small incisions in the skin. The tool then inflates the abdominal cavity using carbon dioxide and allows the surgeon to perform the surgery internally, avoiding large incisions. Used as a primary surgical technique for the removal of gallbladders, laparoscopy is being used more and more in IBD surgeries.

Different conditions call for different surgeries. Some surgeries are minor enough for the patient to walk out of the hospital the same day and others are more life-altering. In this chapter, we will explore the different options that fall short of the creation of an ostomy. The ostomy surgeries and coping with the ostomy will be covered in Month 4.

Stricture dilation

Though this procedure can and often is performed during colonoscopies by gastroenterologists, there are certain occasions when a surgeon may perform this task, usually in CD patients and usually as an outpatient procedure. The surgeon will use an endoscopic tool to enter the GI tract and locate the stricture. A small balloon is placed inside the stricture and inflated, thus stretching the stricture. The balloon is held in place for a short time to hold the stricture open. After that time, the balloon is deflated and withdrawn. In some individuals, this procedure is repeated on a regular basis, in part to avoid further surgery.

In the case of a low rectal or anal stricture that is not complicated by colon cancer, the patient may be sent home with a long, narrow, finger-like instrument known as an anal dilator. Usually used nightly with a lubricant, the dilator is inserted by the patient and held in place for a short time, typically not more than two minutes, before being withdrawn.

Abscess draining

Generally an outpatient procedure for CD patients, the draining of an abscess is performed by a surgeon who will use a long, thin needle and perhaps an endoscopic tool to reach the site of the abscess; other situations call for the needle or a scalpel to pass directly through the skin to lance the abscess. The tool pierces the abscess, allowing pus to drain. The use of antibiotics can help to prevent the abscess from refilling. However, some individuals must have the abscessed portion of the diseased intestines resected.

Fistula debridement

Some fistulas cause little problem at all, others range in their degree of annoyance, and still more are potentially dangerous. When medication fails to close a fistula, the outpatient option of surgical debridement of the fistula remains for CD patients with the complication. With this technique, the surgeon uses a fine instrument to enter the fistula and scrape scar tissue away from

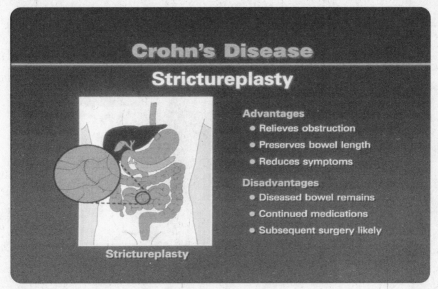

Strictureplasty helps relieve obstructions in some people.
©Crohn's & Colitis Foundation of America (CCFA). Reprinted with permission of CCFA.

the opening and interior of the fistula, allowing the newly agitated tissue to close on its own. For those for whom this technique fails, resection may be the next step. Individuals with internal fistulas such as those that attach different loops of intestines or the intestine and internal organs may only be able to find relief with resection of the diseased loop of intestines and fistulotomy. Also, individuals with rectal fistulas may benefit from an operation that involves cutting a flap into the intestinal wall and pulling the mucosa over the opening of the fistula. The flap is then stitched in place, thus closing the fistula.

Strictureplasty

Generally used in CD patients with tight strictures due to scar tissue, this procedure is like plastic surgery for the intestines. It generally involves a long cut running parallel with the intestines over the affected area. The slit is pinched open in the opposite direction and sewn closed, leaving a slightly shortened but widened opening without losing intestines. Often, this may be the second surgery at the site of a previous resection.

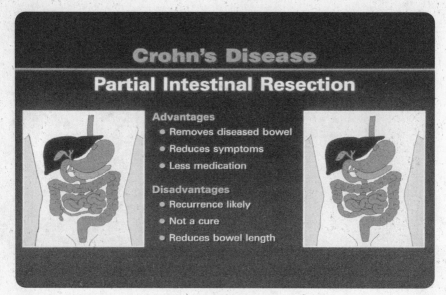

Resection with anastomosis is a relatively common surgery for CD.
©*Crohn's & Colitis Foundation of America (CCFA). Reprinted with permission of CCFA.*

Resection and anastomosis

This surgery goes by a lot of different names and depends on the areas that are being resected and reconnected. For example, an ileocecal resection with **anastomosis** would involve the removal of a diseased segment of the intestines between the ileum and the cecum and the reattachment (anastomosis) of the disease-free portions of the ileum and the cecum. Any resection with anastomosis is used for the removal of an area of intestines causing a hemorrhage, a fistula, a perforated intestine, a stricture, or an obstruction.

Through the use of diagnostic tests such as endoscopy or barium X rays, the surgeon is able to locate the problem area. A disease-free area just before and after the diseased segment is sliced open, freeing the diseased area for removal. The healthy portions are then sewn together again.

In cases where the ileum and colon are attached, it would seem that the larger colon opening would not fit the smaller ileum opening. However, in the case of a stricture or obstruction, the ileum that precedes the stricture often becomes dilated to accommodate the backup of intestinal contents, allowing a good match between the different parts. In other cases, the side of the ileum is attached to the end or side of the ascending colon.

There are a few potential complications with this type of surgery. First, the disease tends to reoccur at the site of the surgery in the months and years following the surgery. Second, a postsurgical abscess can form at the site of the anastomosis. Third, the scar tissue that normally occurs at the site of the anastomosis can shrink and lead to an obstruction.

Ileoanal anastomosis with pouch creation

The reason why this option is separated from the above resection with anastomosis is because it is often used to avoid an ileostomy or colostomy. Also called a pullthrough operation, this surgery calls for the removal of the colon and the reconnection or anastomosis of the ileum with the anus. To facilitate this procedure, the mucosa of the rectum is removed but the outer muscular rectal walls are retained. The ileum is then pulled through the rectum and attached to the anus. With the rectum removed, the reservoir capacity is also removed. To remedy this, a small pouch, called a **J-pouch**, is created from the last foot or so of the ileum.

The entire procedure can be done in one, two, or three operations. In the single operation, the colon is removed, the ileum and anus are connected, and the pouch is created. In the two-stage operation, the colon is removed and the ileum is connected to the abdominal wall in a temporary ileostomy. After a few months, the ileostomy is closed and the pouch is created. In the three-stage operation, the colon is removed, the ileostomy is created, and the rectum remains in place. After a few months, the rectum is removed and the pouch is created, but the ileostomy remains in place to divert the flow of waste and allow the new formation time to heal. The third surgery a few months later unhooks the ileostomy.

In patients with CD, this is not an option as the pouch can become inflamed (**pouchitis**) and would then have to be removed, even if a portion is still healthy. Also, individuals over fifty may not be candidates as the anal sphincter loses muscle tone as the body ages, leading to possible loss of fecal continence.

Aside from pouchitis, the complications that can follow this type of surgery include fecal incontinence, frequent bowel movements, and sexual dysfunction in men.

Bypass

A somewhat common surgical procedure in the past, the **bypass** involved disconnecting diseased portions of the intestine, reconnecting the healthy portions but leaving all parts inside the body. Problems arose when disease activity continued or when cancer formed in the diseased, disconnected segments. Because of this, the segments generally are removed during a surgery.

One fairly rare exception to this happens when the duodenum is diseased and a stricture or obstruction forms. The surgeon then connects the jejunem to the stomach, bypassing the duodenum but leaving it in place. This is done because the duodenum is connected to the mesentery as well as the bile ducts and the pancreas, and is therefore difficult to remove.

Intestinal transplantation

In the relatively middle-aged world of transplantation, this type of surgery is practically a newborn; the first such surgery was performed in 1990. Success rates have slowly climbed since then yet in the twenty-four approved intestinal transplant centers in the United States in 2005, 178 such operations took place.

Candidates for this surgery include CD patients who have had much of their small intestine removed and rely on TPN to receive their nutrition. As liver and septic complications happen to these individuals on occasion, they are left with little choice but to have a cadaveric donor's intestines transplanted into them. Intestinal transplant operations involve a small portion of the bowel such as the small bowel, the entire intestines, or the entire intestines plus the liver.

The majority of the patients who receive this type of transplant are now over the age of eighteen, a very recent development. According to the United Network for Organ Sharing, the one-year success rates for this surgery are about 80 percent, with three-year survival rates closer to sixty percent.

IN A SENTENCE:

> *There are a number of reasons for surgery in UC and CD and options that do not involve an ostomy.*

living

Surviving Surgery and Other Hospital Stays

NO COMPLETELY sane person would want to stay in a hospital for any length of time, but just about everyone who has CD or UC at some point or another will have to endure an overnight or longer hospital stay. Fever, abscesses, surgery, and obstruction are just a few of the reasons a doctor might admit you for treatment or observation. In this month, try to accept that you will be hospitalized at some point in the course of your disease treatment.

Despite their reputation, hospitals are really no place for sick people. Rest is supposed to be a necessity for recovery, but constant interruptions, incessant overhead pages, noisy workers who barge in seemingly at whim and speak in normal or louder tones, roommates who snore at a level that rivals an approaching freight train, and relatives and friends who pop in unexpectedly make the hospital a restless environment. Most likely, at the time of your hospitalization you won't feel well, you may be emotionally rattled, or you might possibly be in pain, making any experience less than enjoyable.

But by making your stay as comfortable and as predictable as possible, you will cut down on the unpleasantness of being in a hospital. Learning right now what you can do to make this possible can make all the difference. It all begins with packing for the experience.

What to bring

When arranging for a planned hospital stay, it helps to draw up a list of the things you will need to bring before packing. Some of the most important items on your list should be toiletries. These everyday items bring a sense of normalcy back into your life. Relying on the hospital to supply them can be a mistake. For example, the hospital can generally come up with shampoo but it is usually not the most desirable kind. I save disposable samples from newspapers or the mail or buy sample sizes from the drugstore. Travel-size portions of toothpaste, mouthwash, and other essentials save room in your bag. Hospitals are dry places, so be sure to bring lip balm and lotion to keep your skin and lips from becoming dry and chapped. (If you arrived at the hospital as an emergency case and did not have time to pack, ask your family members and friends to bring your goods.)

Your own clothing may be a comfort. Bring slippers with nonskid soles and shower shoes. Tops that button up the front tend to be easier to pass an IV bag through the sleeve than pullovers; also, pullovers require the arms to be raised, not a comfortable movement following abdominal surgery. If you plan to have surgery or have a sore abdomen, make sure that the pants or skirts you bring have light elastic waistbands as anything tight or constricting will add to your pain. Never bring valuables such as jewelry, or expensive clothing items such as leather jackets or fur.

Likewise, your own pillow may be a comfort. Personally, I travel with my pillows; I never get the right fit or feeling with institutional pillows in hotels or hospitals. For further nighttime comfort, consider purchasing soft foam ear plugs from a pharmacy, gun shop, or target range to filter out evening noises from the hallways.

For entertainment, hospitals usually supply television at a daily rate; sometimes the selections include a movie channel. If you would like to see a movie not listed, bring a videotape or DVD of the movie with you and request access to a television with a videocassette or DVD player. Many hospitals use this audiovisual equipment for teaching during the day but it is free in the evening. Another option is to bring your own personal device, such as a portable DVD player or an iPod. Also, lightweight reading material is the best for passing time, since you may lack the concentration level to wade through *War and Peace*.

If you regularly consume certain things at certain times of the day such as a bedtime snack or derive comfort from certain food or beverage items, be sure to bring them for when you can resume eating and drinking. Use common sense here. If you drink a glass of wine before retiring every night, it probably isn't a good idea to haul in the rare vintage Chardonnay, a corkscrew, and the crystal. However, pleasantly flavored tea bags, instant hot chocolate, and individually packaged snacks (Rice Krispie Treats, cereal bars, etc.) might provide a respite from bland hospital food. Be sure your doctor approves all goods prior to packing them.

Biding your time in the hospital

Once you are in the hospital, acclimate yourself to your surroundings. Learn about when and what you can eat and drink, what they expect from you regarding the bathroom (sometimes, they want to measure your urinary output and have methods for doing so), how to make phone calls or use the television, and so on. Find out what plans they have for you regarding tests ordered by the doctors, when they will occur and how long they will take. The sooner you know the schedule, the more predictable your stay becomes.

This almost goes without saying, but be nice to your nurses. It goes a long, long way. Ditto for the household staff. During one hospital visit, the woman who mopped the floors admired an arrangement of flowers a friend had given me so I gave them to her. It turned out that she was the one who controlled room assignments and made sure that I had no roommate the last night of my stay.

As for friends and relatives, ask them to call first before visiting to help control the flow of visitors to your room. Also, if you are in a semiprivate room, remember that your roommate might be resting so ask visitors to keep their voices down. Try to keep the visitors on your side of the room as well. Keep visits as long as you feel comfortable and don't feel shy about politely asking them to leave. Don't violate the visiting hours and rules, as it generally makes the staff mad.

Surviving abdominal surgery

Having surgery can be traumatic for anyone, especially the first time. Not knowing what will happen can make you feel powerless to control your destiny as well as your pain. Knowledge about the surgery and the process you will go through afterward can help to lessen the fear and anxiety.

If the surgery is not an emergency, you will have time to prepare. In the days and weeks prior to the surgery, line up any help you need for the time when you are in the hospital and for helping to care for you or your family when you return from the hospital. Frequently, friends, relatives, and neighbors feel helpless to ease your burden. If so, assign them tasks such as preparing meals to have in your freezer for when you return, picking up and caring for children, feeding and caring for pets, taking in mail, etc. It helps to make a list of who is doing what when so no one is duplicating another's tasks.

Your surgeon may put you on nutrition therapy if you are malnourished prior to the surgery. Also, you may have to stop taking steroids, immunosuppressant drugs, and some supplements that may interfere with the healing process or with clotting.

Most surgeons request that the bowel be cleansed the evening before the surgical procedure, likely the night before you leave for the hospital. Generally, this is the same process as a colonoscopy prep (tips found in Month 5) with the addition of multiple doses of erythromycin, a powerful antibiotic that will kill potentially harmful bacteria in the colon. This medication, combined with the bowel cleansing, may make you nauseous; to avoid this, you may want to request that a dose of an antinausea drug like promethazine (Phenergan), trimethobenzamide (Tigan), or ondansetron HCl (Zofran) be available for you.

After checking into the hospital, you may be taken to a preoperative area where you will change into a hospital gown and an intravenous line will be started in your arm. If you are nervous (and who isn't?), ask for something to soothe your anxiety; mild IV sedatives work nicely for this. You may be asked several times as to why you are having surgery and what kind of surgery you are having. Don't be alarmed. They really know why you are there and simply seek to avoid mistakes.

In addition to surgical anesthesia, some surgeons offer an option for epidural pain relief. Like the method used in childbirth, this technique blocks pain you would normally feel following surgery. A quick and relatively painless procedure, it involves a needle inserted into the spinal column that is taped into place. If it works properly and stays in place, you will feel very little to no pain following surgery. When the method is withdrawn, the pain returns, sometimes with surprising intensity. Also, if it slips out of place, you temporarily may not be able to feel or control your lower extremities or you may experience sharp nerve pain or a spinal headache.

When you are finally wheeled into surgery, the doctors will prepare your body by placing surgical draping over the areas that are not to be operated upon. They will position you on the table, placing your arms straight out from the side. The surgeon will then prompt the anesthesiologist to put you under.

When you awake in recovery, the goal is to have you breathe on your own as the nursing staff monitors you for any reactions to anesthesia. Soon, you will be transferred to your regular room to recuperate. When the orderlies do so, remind them to be gentle with you when shifting you from the gurney to your bed. Often, these individuals have never had abdominal surgery and aren't aware of the pain associated with being dumped on a bed.

You may have a urinary catheter inserted. This is to facilitate the drainage of urine since the bladder at times is slow to recover from the effects of the anesthesia. It will be removed as you recover. Other tubes and drains will also be removed as the need for them lessens.

There are a few things you can do to speed your recovery. For one, you will be given a small plastic object with colored balls in it and a small hose attached to it called an incentive spirometer. The doctor will tell you to place your mouth on the hose attachment and suck air from it to raise the balls. By doing this, you will increase your lung capacity and reduce your chances of developing pneumonia, a serious potential postsurgical consequence.

Also, walking soon after surgery may help you to recover more quickly. Make reasonable goals, as doing too much too soon will have the opposite effect. Walking to and from the bathroom can be a good first goal. Making it to the nursing station, then doing one lap down the hall and back, and then two laps is a logical progression. Moving your legs will help to move your bowels, a positive sign that the bowels are once again in working order. If you need assistance in walking, call a nurse or nurse assistant to support you or use your IV pole or railing to lean on.

Pain medication is a wonderful thing when you are recovering, especially directly after surgery or shortly after the epidural is removed. But don't hang on to the medication too long because it can slow the bowels. The sooner you are off the strong stuff and back to the over the counter remedies, the more likely you are to have a bowel movement. If everyone seems to anxiously await the first postoperative bowel movement, it is because its arrival marks the beginning of your bowel's return to normal.

You may notice that doing the smallest things like sneezing or laughing or sitting up can be a painful chore. Likely, the surgeons had to cut certain abdominal muscles to get to the intestines. Those same muscles are associated with a variety of motions such as breathing in sharply to walking, from climbing stairs to driving a car. That doesn't mean that certain accommodations can't be made to ease the pain.

○ Try to relax your belly muscles when sneezing or laughing, compensating with your head, neck, or chest muscles instead.

○ When sitting up from a reclining position, roll onto your side and close to the edge of the bed, swing your legs down, place your arms to the side, and use them to push your torso to an upright position. When all else fails, adjust the hospital bed to a sitting position.

○ Sleeping flat on your back can be uncomfortable for the first two weeks. Place two pillows or a foam wedge draped with a sheet or a towel under your legs. Slowly reduce the height of the prop until your legs are again lying flat.

○ Backaches can occur because the back muscles work with the abdominal muscles for posture; with the abdominal muscles healing, the back muscles have to work twice as hard, causing strained, achy muscles. Use a heating pad or a heat/cold cycle to ease the ache in the back.

○ Avoid clothing that cuts across the incision site, binds, or is tight.

○ When food is reintroduced, take care to chew everything thoroughly and don't be surprised if you feel pain at the site of the surgery. This minor discomfort should ease within the week.

When you are ready to leave, make sure that you have another person there to hear the discharge instructions and request a written copy if you

aren't given one. Also, ask that individual to drop off and pick up any prescriptions for you when you return home.

Be sure to heed the doctor's restrictions regarding activity in the weeks
following surgery. When you are feeling strong enough, ask which activities you can resume. For example, reclaiming my abdominal muscles always
helps me to begin feeling like I am back in my own body. When my surgeon
allows it, I start practicing with the DVD *The Science of Fitness with
Tamilee—I Want That Body!* I do only as much as I can, slowly building back
up to being able to do the abdominal segment of the DVD once a day.

Don't be surprised if your energy doesn't bounce back immediately. Your
body has been through a trauma and it will take time to recover. I promise
that with each passing day you will feel better.

IN A SENTENCE:

> *The hospital is not a patient-friendly place but it and surgery are
> both meant to be survived.*

MONTH **4**

learning

The Ostomy

WITH OTHER IBD surgeries, the essence of bowel function is maintained as the individuals continue to excrete fecal matter through the rectum and anus and into the toilet. But with the ostomy, the waste exits through a hole in the abdominal wall and into a bag or through a tube inserted into an internal reservoir. On the surface, it appears to be another variation of a bowel surgery, but this alteration of bowel function can have greater psychological and lifestyle repercussions than a resection or strictureplasty, for example.

While every attempt is usually made to preserve the integrity of the intestines in IBD medical treatment, sometimes an ostomy is the only or the best choice. The reasons for having an ostomy surgery include:

○ Fulminant colitis and toxic megacolon. With these life-threatening, emergency conditions, a great risk of perforation or hemorrhage exists.

○ Medical treatment failure. Usually not an emergency condition, the ostomy is an option after drug therapy is unable to control the inflammatory process or if scar tissue restricts the colon's ability to function.

○ Colorectal cancer or risk of it. This threat exists for UC and CD patients with long-standing disease in the colon.

○ Fecal incontinence due to rectal stricturing. When the rectum can no longer retain waste in a normal fashion, fecal incontinence can become problematic.

○ Pouchitis or continued fecal incontinence following an ileoanal anastomosis with J-pouch surgery. For fecal incontinence without inflammation, the pouch can be retained and converted into a **Kock pouch** ileostomy, described below.

The preparation of the surgery is the same as is it is for other planned bowel surgery. The patient's nutritional status is brought up to par, steroids and other medications are possibly stopped, and the bowel is cleansed prior to surgery. For emergency surgery, little to no preparation can be done, as waiting for improved nutrition status or cleansing the bowel can pose an additional risk to the patient's condition.

In general, individuals with ostomies have the same kinds of postsurgical risks of infection and bleeding. However, they also carry additional increased risks in the days, months, and years ahead for such things as dehydration and formation of kidney stones due to changes in water absorption, as well as gallstones due to a reduced ability to reabsorb bile salts. The removal of the rectum as well as the body image problems associated with a stoma may affect sexual function in both males and females. A small percentage of males lose their ability to ejaculate or the ejaculate backs up into the bladder as a result of the surgery.

The Kock pouch

There are two main kinds of ostomies, each requiring different circumstances for the patients. One kind is called the Kock pouch or continent ileostomy. Named for the Swedish surgeon who invented the technique, it is used only for UC patients with or without ileoanal anastomosis who have lost or risk losing anal sphincter control, who may have had a **Brooke ileostomy** but want to shed their appliance, or whose job or lifestyle requires them to be away from a toilet but otherwise are candidates for the ileoanal anastomosis. Crohn's patients are not candidates because the procedure requires the formation of an internal pouch with about a foot or

Ulcerative Colitis

Total Colectomy and Continent Ileostomy

Advantages
- Option after standard ileostomy
- Medication rarely needed
- No appliance
- Planned pouch emptying

Disadvantages
- Not for Crohn's
- External stoma
- Possible valve leakage
- Revision sometimes needed
- Limited availability

The Kock pouch is an ostomy alternative for some people.
©Crohn's & Colitis Foundation of America (CCFA). Reprinted with permission of CCFA.

slightly more of the ileum; this poses a risk for future bowel loss if the CD should show up in the pouch. Obese patients and frail patients who would not fare well with potentially more surgery are also not good risk candidates for the surgery.

In this procedure, the surgeon removes the colon and perhaps the rectum and anus. The last foot of the intestines is made into a loop, with the sides touching. The center is stitched together while the top and sides are cut open into one piece. The top is folded down and stitched back to the sides to form a pouch. The end of the ileum is brought to the outside of the abdominal wall below and to the right or left of the belly button where it is changed in shape, called a nipple valve. A drainage tube is inserted into the valve where it will remain for about a month while healing takes place. The rectum and anus are either removed at the time of the initial surgery or are removed at a later date when the patient is better able to withstand the surgery. After a few days, the patient resumes eating, with the intestinal contents draining through the tube.

Following the healing stage, the drainage tube is removed. The patient is then able to drain the pouch with a portable tube that is inserted through the nipple valve and into the pouch. While seated on the toilet, the patient can then slightly press on the pouch to release the contents that then empty into the commode. A small patch can be worn over the valve to absorb leakage of mucous or occasional seepage of pouch contents.

The main advantage of the pouch is that the patient does not have to wear an appliance to catch the waste. The possible complications include all surgery-related complications (infection of site, fever, etc.), as well as incontinence of the pouch, stricture, or obstruction due to scar tissue formation and pouchitis. While the internal pouch may seem very desirable, it is a relatively uncommon procedure and requires a surgeon with special training and skills.

The Brooke ileostomy

Another, more common kind of ostomy surgery is the Brooke ileostomy or incontinent ileostomy. Named for the British surgeon who invented the technique, it is used for either CD or UC patients, specifically individuals with or without ileoanal anastomosis who have lost or risk losing sphincter control, as well as those who may not fare well in a multistage operation. A

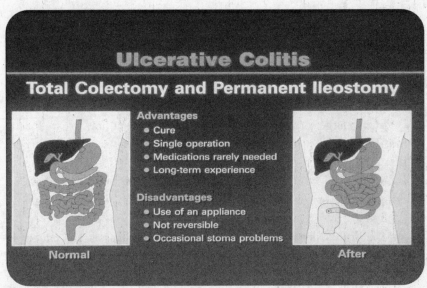

The Brooke ileostomy is considered a cure for UC.

©*Crohn's & Colitis Foundation of America (CCFA). Reprinted with permission of CCFA.*

colostomy also falls into this category as it, too, is not continent and requires the wearing of an appliance.

In this procedure, the surgeon removes the colon and perhaps the rectum and anus; with a colostomy, part of the colon remains. The healthy part of the ileum is then brought to the outside of the abdominal wall below and to the right or left of the belly button. There, the ileum is folded over inside out, like the collar of a turtleneck shirt; the inner mucosa is then fastened to the skin.

Following the surgery, the patient is allowed to begin a clear liquid diet after the stoma begins to discharge waste. This generally takes three to five days. The patient learns to care for the stoma and change the appliance they must wear from then on before they are discharged from the hospital. Over the next few months until total healing occurs, the stoma site is measured in ileostomy or colostomy patients for proper fit of the appliance.

There are very few surgical complications related to this surgery. Those that do occur generally are related to the formation of scar tissue causing stricture or obstruction at the stoma site or the passing of additional intestine through the stoma, called **prolapse**.

The role of the enterostomal therapist

One particularly helpful individual to those undergoing ostomy surgery is the **enterostomal therapist** (ET), usually a specially trained nurse. This individual will likely visit the patient prior to surgery to explain what to expect in terms of postsurgical care and to answer any questions.

Following surgery, the therapist will teach the patient how to care for the stoma. For people with the Kock pouch, the therapist will train them in how to care for the stoma, what potentially worrisome symptoms to look out for, and how to drain the pouch and care for the equipment. Additionally, he or she may offer the patient practical tips on living with the pouch.

For the Brooke ileostomy patient, the therapist will assist the patient in choosing from the many appliances that attach to the body to collect waste. Generally, these come in one- and two-piece units. In the two-piece unit, a face plate is attached to the skin surrounding the stoma, and the plastic bag snaps onto the plate; the one-piece unit contains both the face plate and the bag. The bags are either closed ended or are open at the end to drain and are resealed with a tail clip. Additionally, the therapist will teach the ileostomy patient about the use of adhesives, the care of the skin surrounding the stoma, and any worrisome signs to report to the doctor.

Usually, these individuals are available to the patient through phone calls and other appointments long after the hospital stay is over.

IN A SENTENCE:

> *There are two major kinds of ostomy surgeries, each with its own reasons, benefits, risks, and complications.*

living

Coping with the Ostomy

BECAUSE THE way you go to the bathroom has changed, your life will change in other ways as well when ostomy surgery is performed. Your day-to-day routine will be altered as you learn to change or empty appliances or drain the internal pouch. Sharing the change with others may be awkward or difficult for either party, while others may struggle with facing an intimate occasion for the first time or resuming intimacy in a long-standing relationship.

Although you may never have to have this type of surgery, it is still important to take the time this month to learn about what life will be like if you do eventually have to make this decision or have this decision made for you as it is a possibility in both CD and UC.

Day-to-day changes

For those with colostomy or Brooke ileostomy, one of the first adjustments to be made has to do with wearing the appliance continuously. If you are preparing to have the surgery, it might help to practice by choosing an appliance first and wearing it filled with a little water to find a comfortable spot for the stoma. Learning about the different kinds of appliances and equipment—one piece vs. two pieces, open ended vs. closed ended, skin cleansers, deodorizers, adhesives—may also ease the transition by placing a measure of control in your hands. Most companies offer their supplies in free trial samples. Be sure to take advantage of that service to find the right fit for you.

For those with the Kock pouch, the drainage tube and bag will be an adjustment you will likely have to make immediately following surgery. Realize that this is temporary and that you will soon be using the drainage tube on your own.

Talking to someone who has been through the surgery and successfully lives with an ostomy may also be a comfort. Frequently, enterostomal therapists can connect you with such an individual who lives near you. The United Ostomy Associations of America may also have a chapter near you and can link you up with a fellow ostomate (see information at the end of the chapter). The Internet is also home to many Web boards where questions can be answered and support can be sought.

Following colostomy or Brooke ileostomy surgery, the enterostomal therapist will teach you to either drain the pouch or change the appliance before you leave the hospital. Because many hospital surgical stays can be less than a week, you will most likely be encouraged to phone the therapist with questions and concerns. Some ETs will make house calls.

Emptying the pouch becomes a ritual for Kock pouch patients. Many individuals will have two sets of tubing—one for home and one for away from home. In either case, they are rinsed, patted dry, and kept in a protective sack when not in use. The drainage tubes are small enough to be kept in a purse. Some patients will also carry with them small air freshener sprays to reduce any odor when using a public bathroom.

Similarly, changing the appliance also involves a ritual. Some people keep their supplies in a set location such as a bathroom, a bedroom, or a closet. Usually, they will have tools such as a blow-dryer, scissors, adhesives, and extra appliances in this location at all times. Most individuals with ostomies keep extra supplies with them when they leave the house, usually in a portable satchel or in their purses. The extra supplies mostly come in handy when a seal becomes loose, effluent leaks, or a clip malfunctions.

Rachel, a vibrant sixteen-year-old who underwent a colectomy in December 2000 as a result of toxic megacolon complicating her CD, keeps her supplies in her bedroom. She chose a two-piece, open-ended unit that snaps together like Tupperware.

"When my appliances needs changing, I usually sit down at a little changing station in my room that has all of my ostomy supplies and toiletries near it. I cut another flange and heat it up with a blow-dryer to ensure a better hold. Then I carefully peel off the old flange with the pouch still attached and throw it into a plastic bag. I use stoma paste on the flange but only a little. It helps adhere the flange even better around my stoma. Then after I put on the flange, I snap on a bag, put on a clip and voilà! Brand new bag. There's always something nice about a nice clean appliance," she said. "In my purse I have an emergency pack in case I have a leak or accident when I'm away from home. It includes a flange, a bag, two scissors, a tube of paste, and an extra clip."

Jacy had her routine down pat in two weeks, thanks to an ET who had an ileostomy as well. She carries with her a change of appliance, a collapsible cup for rinsing the bag, and cheap mouthwash, of which she uses about a tablespoon to prevent bag odor. She uses two heavy-duty paper towels and a plastic bag to change and dispose of the bag. "Then it all gets put into a baggie, tied up, and tossed," Jacy says.

Clothing is usually not a problem with a Kock pouch as a slim bandagelike covering can be kept over it to retain any discharge. For a Brooke ileostomy or colostomy, some considerations might be taken to reduce the profile of the appliance. For example, sheer and silky fabrics can show the outline of the appliance more readily than thicker cotton, denim, wool, and blended fabrics. Tighter clothing can be worn, but ostomy patients find that more frequent emptying of their appliance will reduce its profile.

Swimming and other active exercise is also usually not a problem. A waterproof patch or smaller "sport" appliance can be worn beneath a one-piece bathing suits or swim trunks. High-waisted bikinis may also be an option for some. Pleated or patterned suits are best for disguising any unnatural shapes or bulges, and work not only for ostomy patients, but also for people who feel their figures are less than perfect.

Some doctors warn against any contact sports and there is good reason for this, as an appliance can be ruptured. However, some professional athletes, such as the former San Diego Chargers place kicker Rolf Benirschke, have competed while wearing an appliance. It all really depends on how comfortable you feel with the risks.

At work or school, it is helpful to have easy access to a bathroom; in school, having an open-ended bathroom pass is best, and many districts have provisions in place for such an instance. Most likely, you won't be using it as much as you did in the past but emptying your pouch or appliance is likely to happen at least once a day while you are there.

Tom, a UC patient who underwent a colectomy in 1997, keeps a backpack of clothes in his car along with extra supplies in case his two-piece appliance leaks while at work. That way, he can resume his physically demanding job without having to return home to change.

Food is no longer an issue for many ostomates, especially those whose UC was cured with the surgery. Fibrous foods should be avoided or carefully chewed in those who develop a stricture due to CD or scar tissue related to the surgery. Also, seeds and nuts tend to come out whole. Odiferous foods such as asparagus, garlic, onions, and spicy food tend to make for more potent effluent but that is true for everyone. After eating those items, it helps to have some room freshener on hand when the effluent is drained.

Relationships

Broaching the subject of ostomies or ostomy surgery is difficult at best. People are generally just not comfortable about talking about it. Perhaps this attitude can be linked to society's aversion to anything digestive beyond the effect on the palate. The words rectum, anus, or sigmoid rarely enter conversation, and discussion about fecal matter or the process of eliminating waste is considered distasteful. But in some instances, telling individuals about your ostomy is not only helpful but is also unavoidable.

Who you tell about the surgery is entirely dependent upon you. Some individuals prefer to be very open about it, stopping barely short of collaring every stranger on the street and sharing their story. Others keep the information close to the vest, sharing it only with selected, trusted loved ones. Even in work or school situations, often times bosses and teachers are only told the basics, that the person needs to use the bathroom more due to a medical situation.

How much is told is also very personal. Sometimes, the person being told can only grasp the most basic of facts, such as that you need to have a major surgery and will use the bathroom in a different way afterward. Smaller children, for example, are usually happy with that answer. More curious individuals will probably want to know more. How much you tell them goes back to how comfortable you are in sharing that information. Some people will allow others to watch them change an appliance or empty their pouch, but others may feel more comfortable with a stick figure drawing.

For the most part, people are accepting of the information, offering support and understanding. Occasionally, a bad attitude floats to the surface, making those with ostomies seem less human. It is best to ignore such individuals. Rachel came across such an individual on an Internet message board.

"It made me cry but then I realized those people were just ignorant and didn't realize that an ostomy can save someone's life," she said.

For people who have more intimate contact with you, it is usually best to save the medical drama until the relationship is more stable. Developing the emotional component that serves as the binding ingredient in any long-lasting relationship is paramount. Some people may feel that it is hard to be a sex object with a permanent ostomy, but sex—good to outstanding sex, anyway—is about more than physical relations. It is about being emotionally intimate and sharing deeply on many different levels. Therefore, having an ostomy is similar to just about any other physical characteristic like wearing a retainer or eyeglasses.

Coping with this characteristic during intimate moments rarely poses problems. In the Kock pouch patients, a patch can be worn over the stoma. In ileostomy or colostomy patients, a smaller appliance can be worn during those times. Darker lighting and strategically placed clothing can obscure the site as well. Most of all, a lot of confidence and a splash of humor can help you get through any touchy time.

Tom said he has become more adept at the physical side of intimacy since his lifesaving operation. After showering, he uses paper tape to roll up and secure the appliance. "We can have the same kind of intimacy after surgery as we did before the surgery," he said of the relationship he has with his wife. "I think I had a bigger problem than she did after surgery. I am getting better at dealing with it when it comes to sex."

Psychological support

Sometimes, it is hard to get through a time like this on your own. Leaning on friends, relatives, and clergy members can ease the burden for some, but other individuals need a little more outside help in a time like this.

A psychotherapist, especially one specializing in issues surrounding chronic illness, may be of help. For information on locating such an individual, check out the tips in Day 4. Also, the United Ostomy Associations of America exists as a patient education and support organization for individuals who have ostomies of all kinds. Through hundreds of chapters nationwide, the organization offers pre- and postoperative patient support. With this service, the person undergoing the surgery is assigned to a local individual who has undergone special training. The individual will meet with you before and after surgery and be available to you to answer any questions. The organization also offers annual national conferences that boast a number of seminars and social activities for a wide range of participants. Additionally, the organization produces a quarterly magazine for members.

United Ostomy Associations of America, Inc.
P.O. Box 66
Fairview, TN 37062-0066
(800) 826-0826
www.uoaa.org

IN A SENTENCE:

Having an ostomy can affect every area of life but how and to what degree ultimately depends on how an individual handles it.

MONTH5

learning

Cancer
and IBD

FOR THE past few years, awareness of colon cancer occurrence in the general population has risen. There is now National Colorectal Cancer Awareness Month (March), a colored ribbon associated with increased awareness (blue), and major star power behind the cause (Katie Couric).

All of the awareness is needed. Colorectal cancer was diagnosed in 145,290 Americans in 2005, with another 56,290 dying of the disease primarily due to later-stage diagnosis; the deaths accounted for about 10 percent of all cancer deaths in the United States in that year. Though treatments are improving, the key to lowering the death rates is to make sure that individuals have access to and knowledge of timely screening methods.

Aside from age and familial occurrence, one of the major risk factors for developing colon cancer is the presence of IBD. Within this category, further increased risk is associated with the long-term presence of disease activity and the area of involvement of the intestines. Another characteristic that IBD patients share with each other is that the age of onset of the disease is generally one to two decades prior to the onset of the disease in the general population with average risk factors; in other words, the time of diagnosis of colorectal cancer in IBD patients is generally in their forties to fifties, whereas those with average risk factors tend to develop it in their sixties to seventies.

Risk for UC

In the past, scientists have attempted to assess the rate of colorectal cancer occurrence in those who had been diagnosed with UC at least twenty-five years. Different papers released with these criteria pegged the rate anywhere from 3 percent to 42 percent at that given interval. More recent studies have found that the rate of occurrence is closer to 3 to 5 percent eight to ten years after diagnosis, increasing each year thereafter until it is 1 in 5 thirty years after diagnosis.

In general, the greater the extent of the UC, the greater the chance exists of colorectal cancer development. Of UC patients, those with disease that involves the entire colon, pancolitis, are at greater risk than those who have disease located from the descending colon to the rectum and those with disease confined to the sigmoid colon and rectum. However, the cancerous and precancerous lesions tend to be scattered throughout the colon evenly, while colorectal cancer formation in those with no IBD and average risk tend to appear more distally in the sigmoid colon or rectum. Another risk factor appears to be the age of onset of UC. The younger the person at the time of an IBD diagnosis, the greater a chance exists for the later development of cancer.

Another risk factor that bears noting is the presence of the complication of primary sclerosing cholangitis (PSC), a narrowing and stricturing of the biliary system that is prevalent in less than 5 percent of patients with IBD but more often in UC patients than CD patients, and more often in males than females. Not only do these individuals have a greater risk factor for liver and biliary cancer associated with the complication, but they also have higher than normal risk for developing colorectal cancer as well. One medication that seems to mediate this risk in this small population is ursodeoxycholic acid (Urso or Actigall).

Outside of the colorectal and biliary cancer associated with PSC, people with UC and CD also have a higher risk for developing intestinal lymphoma than the general population. Usually, the individual developing this complication will have extensive disease in the colon.

The good news is that the survival rates for colorectal cancer in the UC patient are no different than those of the general population. With proper surveillance as discussed below, UC patients will have a better chance of catching the disease in an earlier stage and thus have better survival chances.

Risk for CD

Up until recent years, the risk of developing IBD-related cancer in Crohn's patients was downplayed. Textbooks would dedicate large sections to colorectal cancer and UC but only a page or two on cancer and CD.

However, researchers recently have paid more attention to the occurrence of colorectal cancer in individuals with Crohn's colitis, saying that the incidence rate is on par with those who have UC. In particular, some studies have reported an elevated risk of developing malignancies in those whose disease was discovered prior to the age of thirty, in those with significant anorectal disease, and in those with colon involvement of the disease for more than eight to ten years.

Despite the fact that most CD occurs in the terminal ileum, negligibly increased rates of small bowel cancers have been reported in CD patients as compared to the general population. One difference in small bowel cancers in CD is that they tend to occur more in the terminal ileum whereas the general population tends to see a more even pattern of distribution.

To a lesser degree than UC patients, PSC remains a threat to a small percentage of CD patients. Because of this, CD patients with PSC share the increased likelihood of developing liver and biliary cancers associated with this condition as well as the increase in colorectal cancers associated. CD patients also share a slightly increased likelihood of developing primary intestinal lymphoma.

Finding the cancerous or precancerous lesions

Doctors and researchers are often like police investigators. If a detective is aware that a potential threat to human life exists, they will watch out for that risk to pop up and nab it before it can do harm. In the same way, IBD doctors like gastroenterologists should be aware that there is an increased risk in IBD patients for developing cancer in certain situations. They should institute a plan to watch out for the early cellular changes that signal possible cancer growth and excise the cancerous tissue at the earliest possible chance.

There is a little controversy surrounding the timetable for the beginning and scheduling of surveillance, with some saying annual surveillance should begin eight years after diagnosis and others saying a complete examination every five years would be less stringent yet effective. But most agree that the best way to find the cancer in an IBD patient is through the use of the colonoscopy rather than the barium enema or virtual colonoscopy. Part of the reason for this is that many who develop colorectal cancer in IBD have cancers that appear as flat, plaque-like lesions, as opposed to more prominent polyps that more easily appear on such an X-ray or scan. Aside from the fact that the colonoscopy allows the doctor to actually see the bowel walls, the endoscopic tool allows the doctor to take numerous biopsies of tissues that can be later examined for the presence of precancerous cellular changes called **dysplasia.**

Dysplasia is another point of controversy in IBD occurrence of colon cancer. Technically, this is the presence of cellular changes within the mucosa that usually heralds the formation of colorectal cancers. In the low-grade form, a number of cellular changes can be seen within the cells themselves as well as within the structure of the epithelium, such as crypts branching out and enlarging. In high grade dysplasia, the changes are more severe both within the cells and within the structure of the epithelium. Some pathologists differ in their definitions of what is high grade and what is low grade.

When doctors take biopsies, the pathologist must then determine the status of the sample, whether it has dysplasia or not or, if it is indefinite. In the case of a negative sample, the controversy pretty much stops there. With an indefinite diagnosis, they must try to determine if the sample is possibly negative, unknown, or possibly positive. With a positive sample, they must determine if the piece they are examining is high or low grade dysplasia, a tricky definition for some to ascertain. It is further complicated if disease activity is present, and by the fact that it can happen in several locations within the colon and rectum.

And the controversy is not over. The vast majority of doctors agree that if high-grade dysplasia is present, the patient should probably undergo a proctocolectomy before cancer forms. The group, however, diverges on the treatment plan for individuals with low-grade dysplasia. Some have noted that it occasionally recedes while others find that it is simply a precursor to high-grade dysplasia, the step before cancer formation. In general, more frequent colonoscopies are performed to monitor the situation, with a proctocolectomy performed at the appearance of high-grade dysplasia; however, some doctors prefer to recommend proctocolectomy with low-grade dysplasia, as these tend to be markers for high-grade dysplasia as well. In this case, it pays to get a second or third opinion before undergoing surgery.

If regular surveillance fails to catch the appearance of cancer or if surveillance is not done and cancer appears, most likely a proctocolectomy will be performed and the excised colon will be examined by the pathologist. The tumor is then "staged," meaning that its spread will be determined and the cancer will be categorized into one of several groups. Treatment is generally determined by the stage of the cancer.

Prevention

Prevention of cancer in the IBD patient is one of the keys to long-term survival and the greatest tool a patient has is the participation in a regular surveillance program. Although you are only five months from your diagnosis, there are some things that can be done now by you and your doctor. For example, the doctor should assess the patient's risks by asking about other risk factors, such as the colon cancer incidence rate within your close relatives and personal habits such as smoking (smoking was recently discovered to be a possible risk factor for the formation of colon cancer). He or she should then lay out a plan for monitoring the presence of cellular changes with a colonoscopy or sigmoidoscopy, such as when it should begin and how often it will occur.

There has been some study in recent years about the effect of diets rich in folic acid, calcium, and vitamin D on the formation of colon cancer. The jury is still out on the findings, but early results suggest that individuals who lack such substances in their diets had a much higher risk of developing colon cancer.

In IBD, it may be logical to think that individuals on sulfasalazine, which tends to block folic acid absorption, would be at greater risk for colon cancer development, since the general science indicates that those who lack folic acid tend to have higher rates of colon cancer. However, some studies indicate that those who use sulfasalazine, mesalamine, and balsalazide tend to have lower rates of colon cancer. At the same time, people with CD in the ileum may need calcium supplementation due to malabsorption of this mineral during flare-ups, not only to protect against osteoporosis but also to potentially protect against colon cancer. A discussion with a doctor about supplementation may be helpful.

As always, a healthy diet rich in fruits, vegetables, lean protein, and grains combined with exercise has been shown to decrease general cancer risk in all individuals, as has avoiding risky behavior such as smoking or being overweight or obese.

IN A SENTENCE:

> *An increased risk of colon cancer exists in both UC and CD patients with long-standing disease of the colon, and regular screening can be used to monitor the possible development of precancerous lesions.*

living

Surviving the Colonoscopy Prep and Other Awful Tests

LIVING WITH IBD will most likely mean having to undergo some of the most wretched tests invented by man. You will have to swallow a pulverized, suspended form of a rock or a dirty dishwater tasting drink, or have a tube snaked through an area clearly marked "exit only." While you don't have to like the procedures, you can learn to live with them through a few simple tips that you will learn this month in the following pages.

The ranking of these tests is based on personal experience. Not everyone will rank these the same.

DEXA scan

Perhaps the easiest of all tests is one that is done the least often, the DEXA (dual X-ray absoptiometry) scan to measure bone density. There is no special diet to follow, no prep to swallow, and patients can usually wear their own clothing. The scan is done to individuals who are on corticosteroids and are at risk of bone density loss.

The patients recline on a padded table for a few minutes as the scan measures the density of some of the larger bones in the body. After the test, the patients simply leave and later contact their doctors for the results.

Ultrasound

The next easiest test for IBD patients is the ultrasound. For this test, there usually is no diet to follow except in the case of the suspicion of gallstones where some patients will refrain from eating for several hours before the test. Scheduling this test first thing in the morning when there is food restriction involved usually makes the fast easier. In addition to ruling out gallstones, the test is done to locate an abscess in an individual who can't tolerate a CT scan.

Again, the patient reclines on a padded table or bed for a few short minutes. The patient may be asked to change into a hospital gown or surgical scrubs to avoid soiling clothing with the gel that is used, and to allow for greater access. If your hospital has patient comfort in the forefront, they will usually have a bottle warmer for the gel that is swathed over the belly before the ultrasound wand is used. If not, the coldness of the gel may be a breathtaking shock and will surely be the most discomfort you will experience during the test.

The technician will then guide the wand over the belly in search of different anatomical structures, pressing gently to obtain a better shot that will appear in grainy black and white on a computer monitor. They will then press a button to secure the image and print it out. The test is usually completed in a few minutes, after which you should be given a towel to wipe off the gel. After getting dressed, you are allowed to leave. Be sure to call the doctor later for the results.

CT scan

Also called the CAT scan or computerized tomography, this test is used in cases where an abscess or hemorrhage is suspected or when a patient may have an obstruction but would not tolerate a small bowel barium series. It is also used in some cases prior to surgery to aid the surgeon in determining anatomical structures such as the location of ureters.

The CT scan may involve a fast of four to six hours prior to the test time, but I have had this test on an emergency basis where no prep was followed. If fasting is called for, scheduling the test in the early morning will take the edge off any hunger. The CT scan will usually involve the injection of a contrast solution. It may also involve the ingestion of several ounces of a clear liquid that can be best described as tasting like weak or dirty dish-water. Swallowing yucky things has never been my forte, especially swallowing yucky things while dressed in a hospital gown in the ER at 1 A.M. But the best way I have found to do so is not to sip it, but rather to drink it as fast as possible. Don't plug your nose as the lack of breathing can heighten the gag reflex, which is probably working overtime from the split second that the fluid touches the palate. Other techniques I use include pacing the hall after swallowing to avoid throwing the liquid up, or sucking on a hard lemon candy to disguise the taste.

If all else fails and you can't keep the fluid down, a nurse or nurse assistant will place a nasogastric tube up your nose and down your throat and slowly inject the fluid into the tube. An NG tube is not a pleasant option, but can be made less painless by sucking water through a straw at the time that the tube is being inserted or with the use of throat numbing spray. When those options are not available, realize that the tube takes seconds to place and the discomfort will be over with soon.

The test requires the patient to recline on a table that will slowly slide into an open-ended cylinder. The machine then makes several clicking noises as X rays are being taken in a circular fashion. If you are claustrophobic or uncomfortable, you can ask that a sedative be placed in the IV line. The test ranges in length but can last about an hour in some cases. After the test, the IV will be withdrawn and you can call the doctor later for results.

Small-bowel series

Otherwise known as the barium swallow, this test is used to locate and determine the activity of CD in the small bowel. It can be helpful in determining the narrowness of a stricture and may point to the presence of a fistula or abscess as well.

The patient usually fasts six to eight hours before the test. It might be easiest to schedule this test first thing in the morning so that you are not overcome with hunger. The worst part about the test for nearly everyone is the taste of the barium, a white, thick, chalky tasting substance made from a pulverized rock suspended in liquid. While food researchers have been able to morph soybeans into delicious meat-like products, and we have been able to accomplish space travel and other spectacular feats of science, the taste of the barium has never been changed. I believe that whoever is able to make it taste like a Häagen-Dazs milkshake should certainly win the Nobel Prize for medicine. Since that hasn't happened so far in my lifetime, the previous tips for swallowing yucky things apply here.

The test may involve an examination of the stomach in which case it begins with the swallowing of about a shot glass portion of strawberry-flavored fizzy liquid that will make you feel as if you have to belch. Don't. This is quickly chased with a very heavy small glass of barium to coat the intestines. You may then be vigorously shaken and rolled about on the table to coat the stomach before X-rays are taken. You will have to drink a few more glasses of barium after the initial X-rays are taken. As the liquid wends its way through the intestines, more X-rays are taken to highlight different intestinal loops. At the end, the ileum may need to be separated to highlight certain segments. The technician will place a paddle with a ball attached to it onto your stomach to gently but firmly separate those loops. This can hurt, especially if you are particularly tender in that spot. I assure you that this will be over quickly.

After you are done, you may be instructed to drink a small portion of milk of magnesia to help move the barium through. You can then get dressed and leave. Don't be alarmed if in the coming days you pass white fecal matter. This is barium.

Colonoscopy

The colonoscopy is a very versatile and useful procedure that is used for many purposes including examining for cancer, locating and excising polyps, and securing biopsies that can be later examined for CD or UC. In the past, it was done on patients who were fully awake, but less unpleasant methods are used now, leaving most patients to ask if the procedure has started when it is already done.

As you probably have heard, the worst part is the prep, an amazing statement given that there are at least a half a dozen ways that the prep is done. The goal of the preps is to strip away any fecal matter from the intestines, thus thoroughly cleansing the intestinal walls for a better view for the endoscopist. All of the preps involve ingesting a substance that then causes intense peristaltic waves and quick evacuation of the bowels, usually taking one to three hours.

Perhaps one of the older preparation ways is the use of a product called Go-Litely, which should probably be named Go Hard and Hurtfully. This involves drinking a glass of barely palatable salty liquid every few minutes until the only thing coming out of you resembles water; a gallon is the usual amount prescribed. A variation of that is Nu-Litely, a less salty, less cumbersome, but no more palatable concoction that works in the same manner. Some doctors prescribe different mixes of castor oil, citrate magnesium, Dulcolax tablets or suppositories, and Fleet enemas to be taken at various times in the two days leading up to the big day. Another product is Fleet Phosphosoda, an intensely briny-tasting liquid. The label says that the patient can mix three tablespoons of the liquid with three ounces of water; for a usual colonoscopy prep, a dose the night before and another the morning of the test usually does the trick. The X-ray prep is similar in that it involves drinking about two doses of two ounces of the nasty tasting prep liquid. Finally, the newest prep, allow the patient to skip the bad taste by swallowing pills chased with an eight-ounce glass of clear liquid; these are commonly known as Visicol or OsmoPrep. On the day before and the morning of the test, the patient has to swallow three to four pills every fifteen minutes over the period of an hour; the total number of pills swallowed each time is eighteen to twenty.

There are drawbacks to every prep, chiefly swallowing things that will make you feel queasy. Because this prep is primarily done at home there are a few things you can do to make it more comfortable for yourself. Remember, these are tips and suggestions; I am not a doctor, and although I have survived this test more times than any doctor I know, you should always follow the directives that your doctor gives to you regarding medication and bowel cleansing solutions.

We'll start with a shopping list. Since you will be headed to the store to pick up the bottles and boxes of prep materials, pick up the following, as you will need them if you don't already have them:

1. Kleenex brand Cottonelle toilet paper infused with both aloe and vitamin E or a box of baby wipes infused with aloe (the quilted wipes provide that extra degree of comfort but may not be advisable if you have a septic system).
2. Hemorrhoidal cream such as Anusol HC or any other one with HC on the label. The HC stands for hydrocortisone, a topical steroid that helps reduce swelling and itching.
3. K-Y Jelly or Vaseline.
4. Plenty of reading material. I prefer to read tabloids that I never read otherwise, as it certainly provides a diversion. I pick up such paragons of journalism as *The National Enquirer, The Star, The Sun,* or the *Weekly World News.* Any other reading material that you would consider fun or distracting is a plus here as well.
5. Scented candles or fragrant bath oil in a pleasing, relaxing scent.
6. A heating pad or hot water bottle.
7. Lots of your favorite clear liquid or semi-liquid food items (avoid all with red or purple dyes as the dye can be mistaken for inflamma- tion), such as ginger ale, Jell-O, Italian ice, popsicles, and chicken or beef broth. Also, be sure to pick up some liquids containing elec- trolytes such as Gatorade or Pedialyte.

First, I have a little rule that whatever goes in must come out, kind of like Newton's law but with a little digestive twist—call it Jill's law. The older preps used to dictate a diet devoid of roughage and fat followed for three days before the test, with a clear liquid diet on the last day. Why? Because these things tend to stay in the colon the longest. With less in there, it made the prep a little easier. People were told to eat baked chicken, baked fish, or scrambled egg whites for protein; less than two tablespoons of oils or fats for the whole day, which meant no cheese, egg yolks, or fried foods; doses of soluble fiber such as plain pasta, white rice, baked potatoes, and white bread; sweets like angel food cake or vanilla wafers; and plenty of clear liquids such as broth, weak tea or coffee without cream, soda pop, and clear juices such as apple juice or white grape juice. The last part, the clear liquids, was all a person could consume the day before. But some doc- tors theorized that the newer preps could do the job without the diet, still stripping everything in their path.

However, I still believe in the old diet. As someone who has had more colonoscopies than I care to remember, the diet helps to eliminate the bulk of the feces prior to prep, leaving less to evacuate. It also makes the liquid fast easier to tolerate for me. I also add a Dulcolax tablet two nights before the blessed event to help get some of the heavy lifting out of the way first. My feeling is that if I can get the prep done in one dose, I have eliminated some of the misery. I also add clear electrolyte beverages like Gatorade or Pedialyte to the diet, sipping them almost constantly in the two days before the test. This will help to boost some of your electrolyte levels as many electrolytes are lost during the prep, leaving some people to feel cold, shaky, and faint. I am not a fan of Gatorade, but I love the Pedialyte because it tastes almost like Kool-Aid. I mix a bit of the orange flavor with ginger ale and crushed ice, a precolonoscopy cocktail.

For swallowing the nasty prep liquids, the rules for swallowing yucky things apply again, only this time, you may have more options than you do in a hospital setting. With the Go-Litely and Nu-Litely, you can add a little Crystal Lite for a bit of flavor. Lemons or limes dipped in sugar and tucked into the cheek counterbalance the salty flavor as well as can hard candy. With the Fleet Phosphosoda, 7-Up, ginger ale, Sprite, or apple juice can be substituted for the water; when I used to do this prep, I drank Sprite, but be forewarned that you may not look at these liquids in quite the same manner in the future. Some people also swear by having the liquid as cold as possible. If you do this, be aware that you might have a sudden, sharp headache more commonly known as brain freeze.

Do not stray too far from the bathroom. In fact, have it as stocked as it can be. You will need K-Y Jelly or Vaseline, the hemorrhoidal cream, the special toilet paper or baby wipes, reading material, bedtime clothing, a bath towel, the aromatherapy tools, and anything else you can think of to add to your comfort. One friend of mine hauls in her television for the event.

You may feel somewhat nauseous and this is natural. Use cold cloths on your forehead or splash cold water on your face to fend off vomiting. Pacing helps as well, but don't go too far from the bathroom, because soon you will have an urge to go that you have never known before.

Before you begin to empty out, it helps a bit to coat your anus with the K-Y Jelly or Vaseline. The velocity at which your intestinal contents exit paired with the volume of the intestinal contents, and the fact that some unabsorbed digestive enzymes will find their way out, can make for a very sore anus and rectum. To ward this off a bit, it helps to thoroughly coat the anus and anal canal with the petroleum products. As the emptying begins, use the gentle wipes and flush often.

As the bowel evacuation subsides, you may feel cold and weak with muscle cramps. At this time, I usually draw a hot bath filled with scented bath crystals or oils and surround it with scented candles. This is soothing. If I still feel the urge to go, I am two steps from the toilet and a bath towel is always nearby. Before getting into my nightgown, I use a little soothing hemorrhoidal cream.

Following the first part of the prep, most doctors allow their patients to continue drinking clear liquids until midnight. This is important, as the bowel-cleanse solutions often draw water from the body into the intestines, causing diarrhea during the evacuation process. This can make you dehydrated. Try to shoot for at least 24 ounces if you can.

On the day of the test, you will be asked to disrobe. Women may have to take a pregnancy test. An IV will be inserted in your arm before you are wheeled into the endoscopy suite. Draping will cover your body and your doctor will place a sedative in your IV. Usually, the painkiller Demerol is used with the sedative Valium and Versed, a short-term amnesia drug. Another option is to use a short-term anesthesia, administered by an anesthesiologist. While you are out, your doctor will insert the endoscopic tool and examine the colon, taking biopsies as well.

The next thing you should remember is waking up in recovery. You may be given juice to drink. When you are able to stand up, you can get dressed. The doctor who performed the test will discuss his or her findings with you and with the person who drove you to the test before you are allowed to leave. You may be woozy the rest of the day but you should recover by the next day.

If you experience sharp pain or a lot of bleeding, you should call the doctor. Rarely, a perforation of the intestines can occur.

Barium enema

This test is used for diagnostic purposes as well as to check for some colon cancers when a scope can't get past a stricture. It can be useful in diagnosing a fistula or a stricture as well.

The reason I rank this test as the worst is that you have to go through the colonoscopy prep but instead of not remembering the test, you stay awake while a large amount of barium and possibly air is inserted through the anus while different X-rays are taken in different positions on a table that moves—hardly a trip to Disneyland for me.

The tips for the colonoscopy prep apply here. The best way to get through the test is to try to relax the stomach, rectal, and anal muscles as much as possible. The enema tip is inserted into the anus and held in place by a gentle but firm tape; a variety of X-rays are then taken. The process takes about twenty minutes in total, longer with a less experienced technician.

When finished, the enema tip is withdrawn and you are allowed to use the bathroom. Also, a dose of milk of magnesia will help some of the barium to move through. Again, don't be alarmed by the white feces; it is barium.

In the future

You may have read about the new pill-shaped camera that can be swallowed or the diagnostic possibilities of the "virtual colonoscopy," a CT scan of the colon using air to inflate the intestine that produces two- or three-dimensional images. While these are significant advances, one must also realize that they do not spare the colonoscopy as tissue samples are important for diagnosis. Neither of these are widely available and probably won't be for at least a decade.

IN A SENTENCE:

> Tests for IBD can be arduous but endurable by following a few suggestions.

MONTH 6

Sex and Fertility

SEX IS everywhere. It invades movies even when the plot has nothing to do with sex. In television series, it is usually part of the plot of a season finale. In advertising, it seeps into everything from motor oil ads to Diet Coke commercials. The covers of women's magazines proclaim articles that hold the keys to tempting any man in five easy steps, while men's magazines give recipes for libido-enhancing concoctions. Aside from the media influence, sex and sexual relationships dominate our culture, as ours is a couples-based culture, and the two halves of a couple are usually assumed to be having sex with one another.

Let it be stressed that, for the most part, individuals with CD and UC lead normal, healthy sex lives. But let it also be said that sex, fertility, and diarrhea do not always go hand in hand—at least not easily. And that is where some people with IBD run into problems, something you may have noticed already. Since IBD occurs in people of all ages, the effects on sexuality and fertility will be wide ranging. While the twentysomething bride may fret over whether or not she will be able to be able to conceive, the fiftysomething man may be more worried about maintaining an erection. Similarly, a preteen girl (hopefully) won't bemoan the fear of incontinence during intercourse, but she may complain that she is not menstruating yet like her peers. As such, the impact on the individual will vary greatly from person to person and from age to age.

The physical and emotional effects

Much of what we feel regarding the physical effects of the disease can and does enter our most intimate relationships on some level. Physically, fatigue and pain—together or alone—are two things that can put the damper on anyone's sex drive. Commonly, these two characteristics are present with disease activity, making sex a low priority at times. Anemia that causes the fatigue can be particularly draining, making sleep and rest seem more desirable than intercourse. At the same time, the pain associated with an inflamed gut can be distracting and an especially big turn off, particularly if the pain is in the rectum. Rectal fistulas and abscesses may be temporary, painfully obvious obstacles to sexual fulfillment in some. Surgical pain, particularly following abdominal surgery, can delay intimacy until an individual is fully healed.

A few individuals who have undergone ostomy surgery also may experience a rare complication when the nerve that controls ejaculation and erection is damaged or severed during the surgery. This makes maintaining an erection or having normal ejaculation impossible in some. For women, the surgery leaves a void in the abdominal cavity, at times allowing the uterus to settle further backward. This change can bring about pain upon intercourse.

The same is true of the emotional effect of the disease. Emotionally, the impact of the diseases can weigh heavily enough to affect sexuality. For one, the depression that can follow diagnosis or reemerge during a recurrence of symptoms may leave an individual feeling less amorous. Medications to treat the depression, such as Prozac, can further complicate the problem, as a diminished libido is one of the medication's side effects.

Fears related to disease activity can also cool things off. In particular, fears of fecal incontinence during intercourse can keep some from even starting. Also, some individuals may have experienced pain during or following intercourse that leads them to be a bit shy the next time the opportunity arises.

Surgical scars, ostomies, and physical changes due to medication or extraintestinal manifestations of the disease may not be physically painful, but may have an emotional toll on sexual intimacy because they may have a negative impact on body image. Some individuals find that these changes make them feel less confident about their bodies and thus less attractive in the eyes of others, further leading them to avoid any sexual situations.

The healthy partners may be keenly aware of this physical and emotional struggle as well. At times, they may feel they have played a part in pain that results from intercourse. As a result, they may be inhibited from pursuing sexual relations with their IBD-affected loved ones.

Fertility and IBD

One concern of both doctors and patients alike is the effect of the disease on fertility. Part of the reason for this is that the largest portion of patients are younger than thirty-five when they are diagnosed, a time when they are either looking forward to their reproductive years or are in the midst of them.

For UC patients, the good news is that fertility is generally unaffected by the disease. Even in CD patients, fertility is only slightly lowered, happening in women largely when disease activity is at its highest. Aside from the physical or emotional effects of the disease that may limit sexual activity, one theory for the lessened fertility is that the fallopian tube may be blocked by inflammation, thus causing a barrier for the ova.

For men in general, lessened sperm count and mobility has been associated with the drug sulfasalazine. By reducing the dose or switching to a 5-ASA drug such as Pentasa or Asacol, the sperm suppression usually resolves, and counts and mobility are increased.

IN A SENTENCE:

> *Certain developments in IBD can put a damper on one's sex life.*

living

Intimacy Issues

SOMEHOW, IT doesn't seem fair that the diseases that affect our digestive system so thoroughly, that suck the joy out of eating, that affect the far reaches of the body from the skin to the major organs, can also have a devastating effect on our sexuality. But life isn't always fair or just and, thus, sex can be affected by the diseases. However, how you deal with those effects will determine just how fulfilling your sex life will be.

When and what to tell

One of the major struggles that individuals with IBD have in telling others occurs in the single person. When and how to tell someone new about the disease is a difficult process when the potential for sex isn't involved, more so when the possibility of an intimate encounter exists. You probably shouldn't do this by hauling your potential mate off to a support meeting on the first date. A good time to do this is after a solid emotional relationship has formed and when sex is not in the immediate offing. Waiting to tell a person that you have an inflammatory condition that causes diarrhea or resulted in an ostomy right as you are ripping each other's clothes off is probably not a great idea either. Instead, pick a less sexually charged time and place.

At first, you may want to tell them the basics such as what the disease entails and how it affects your daily life. Spare them the gruesome details until they are ready for more information. This, of course, may never happen. My husband, for example, decided not long after I was diagnosed that he didn't want to know more—and he is the son of a gastroenterologist! In his case, ignorance is bliss. But if your partner wants more information, direct him or her to books or websites with which you are familiar. Be open to answering any questions they may have as well.

Continuing the conversation after physical intimacy initiates will help to keep the door open for other questions and concerns that arise. In times when the disease is in remission, there may be little discussion about its effect. Conversely, there may be more discussion and concern when the disease is active. This is especially true if your partner thinks he or she is causing you pain during intimate moments or if sex is just not in the picture on a particular night. Assuring them that they are not the root of the problem may spare some difficult feelings. This open line of communication serves as a basis of trust, a key element in any long-term, successful relationship.

Adjusting to situations

Still, problems may continue to exist. Let's face it—it is hard to be in the mood if you have to run into the bathroom. Emily knows a little about this. She and her husband have a healthy, normal sex life, but when her CD is active, she struggles to keep up.

"When the disease is active, it's like I'm so in tune with the inner workings of my digestive system that the sex drive just kind of drops off the radar screen. It's hard to feel sexy when you can feel your dinner moving through your large intestine!" she said.

Even when the drive is there, the diseases can require a few adjustments. Sometimes, intercourse may be too painful or arduous. And other times, nature calls a little too strongly and insistently in the middle of the best part.

How you handle these moments will influence how your partner handles them. Lynn has a healthy sex life but there are times when she just feels too lousy to be much of a sexual force to contend with in the bedroom. On other occasions when her CD is flaring, she feels more vaginal pain and has less bowel control. This could potentially spell disaster, but she and her husband take things in stride or even find humor in the moment.

"Sex has been interesting with this disease to say the least," she said. "It has been a learning experience."

"I tend to have more pain vaginally during this time than during other times. I also have to stop having sex to go to the bathroom sometimes too and that is embarrassing. We now just grin and bear it," she said. "Sometimes the pressure can be too much and accidents do happen. We usually giggle about them."

Finding the solution to the issue depends on how open, diligent, and creative the couple can be. There are plenty of ways to be intimate outside of intercourse. From oral sex to hugging, from a rapturous make out session to the use of sex toys, from mutual masturbation to cuddling, the options run the gamut. Trying something new involves a lot of trust and willingness, but can be very rewarding.

If problems continue to persist despite the best of attempts, a couples or sex therapist can usually help. Again, willingness on the part of both partners is important. To find out how to locate a therapist, see Day 4.

IN A SENTENCE:

> *Maintaining a healthy sex life is possible, even when illness is present.*

HALF-YEAR MILESTONE

You are now through the first half of the first year since diagnosis. As you continue on your journey you have:

○ LEARNED THE IMPORTANCE OF NUTRITION IN MAINTAINING HEALTH AND AS A TREATMENT IN SOME CASES;

○ REALIZED THAT THERE ARE A NUMBER OF SURGICAL PROCEDURES TO TREAT THE CONDITIONS FOR A VARIETY OF REASONS;

○ DISCOVERED TIPS AND SUGGESTIONS FOR MAKING ROUTINE TESTS MORE ENDURABLE; AND

○ FOUND THAT A COLORECTAL CANCER RISK EXISTS FOR PEOPLE WHO HAVE HAD THE DISEASES UNDER CERTAIN CONDITIONS.

Pregnancy, Childbirth, and Lactation

PLANNING A pregnancy can be among life's greatest joys. This expectation of new life paired with the creation of a legacy brings promise for the future and the creation of a new family generation to celebrate.

Pregnancy and childbirth are not only possible for IBD patients, they are expected in many cases. Because the majority of IBD cases are diagnosed either during or before reproductive years, the effect of the diseases and treatments on pregnancy, childbirth, and lactation is a very important subject for physicians and patients, both male and female. Preferably, a frank discussion between the patient and the physician will occur before conception takes place so decisions can be made regarding treatment options ahead of time.

Preparation is key

Planning a healthy pregnancy is the key to reducing the amount and kind of maternal and fetal complications. All women considering pregnancy, for example, should stop smoking and take prenatal vitamins to reduce the chances of such things as low birth weight and neural tube birth defects. In IBD, the preparation and planning for pregnancy is of paramount importance since studies show that one third of pregnant patients will experience a worsening of symptoms, one third will have their symptoms remain as they currently are throughout the nine months, and another third will have an improvement in symptoms. As a rule, those who are in remission will most likely remain in remission and have the fewest number of complications during their pregnancy. In other words, the healthier the patient is, the healthier the pregnancy and the child will be. For those with active disease at the time of conception, the chances are greater that the pregnancy will end in stillbirth or spontaneous abortion. Also, those with active disease risk having a child who is small for gestational age, low birth weight, or delivered earlier than those who are healthy.

For men with IBD, the issue of planning becomes important in the choice of medications that are used not only at the time of conception but in the three months prior to conceiving. Taking sulfasalazine, for example, may result in a lower sperm count, as discussed in Month 6. There is also some controversy provoking findings that taking immunosuppressive drugs such as 6-MP or azathioprine (Azasan, Imuran) in the three months prior to conception may cause complications with fetal health; a handful of smaller studies document the occurrence of higher numbers of newborn abnormalities and spontaneous abortions in cases where the father was taking 6-MP or azathioprine, compared to lower numbers in cases where the father was not taking those medications. Doctors and researchers continue to debate these findings.

Because of the effect of the diseases on maternal and fetal health, medication and medical treatment becomes increasingly important to those planning pregnancy or currently pregnant, whether planned or unexpected. While many women would like to experience a pregnancy taking nothing more than a daily vitamin, those with IBD fare better if the inflammation is controlled during the pregnancy through the use of medication.

I can't stress enough the importance of learning as much as possible about the potential side effects on the fetus or child in choosing to take or not take certain medication. Do not make any decisions until you personally have weighed all of the evidence and feel comfortable with the path you are taking.

Medication and the effect on fetal health

Embryonic and fetal exposure to medication in utero can have an impact on the normal formation that ranges from mild to severe. Exposure that occurs in the first two weeks following conception will either result in the loss of the embryo or the embryo will patch up the damage and continue to develop. In the next ten to twelve weeks, exposure to harmful substances can impair the normal development of the internal organs and can again result in the loss of the pregnancy. Many, many pregnancies are lost during this time for a variety of reasons, not all due to medication. Following this first trimester, exposures to harmful substances can still cause damage to the developing brain and can result in behavioral or growth issues in the years to come. It should be noted that even in the healthiest patients in the general population, abnormalities in gestation and in infants are found. In fact, every pregnancy carries between a three and five percent risk for birth defects.

It is important to know, then, which medications have the potential for damage and which are considered safe. Because of this, a Food and Drug Administration rating system of medication and their potential for teratogenic effect or negative impact on the developing fetus was created. This system ranks the drugs by letter grade with A being a category of drugs proven to have no negative effect through X, drugs that have clear abortive effects or cause severe congenital malformations.

Perhaps the most common medications that patients with IBD are prescribed are the aminosalicylates, including sulfasalazine. That is because these are considered appropriate medications for UC patients and for some CD patients with disease from the ileum through the colon who have mild to moderate disease or for those trying to maintain remission. These medications include Canasa suppositories and Rowasa enemas, as well as Pentasa, Asacol, Colazal, and Dipentum tablets and capsules.

With sulfasalazine, initial reports indicated a possible increase in congenital deformities for the children of parents who were on the medication at the time of conception. However, other, larger studies since then have revealed more positive findings, including one large study in which the children of patients taking sulfasalazine at the time of conception had fewer congenital deformities than children of parents not taking the medication. Most of these drugs are rated in the B category, meaning that there is currently no established relationship between exposure and resulting congenital malformations; only olsalazine (Dipentum) is rated category C.

Other 5-ASA preparations have not been studied as thoroughly, in part because they are newer medications. However, because of the low amount of systemic absorption of the medication, it is routinely believed that the use of the medication is safe during pregnancy. One Canadian study matched 165 women exposed to 5-ASA preparations during pregnancy with another similarly sized group of women who had no such exposure. There were a slightly lower reported number of congenital deformities in the children born to the 5-ASA group than in the control group, and there were no differences in spontaneous abortions, stillbirths, or delivery methods. Where the 5-ASA group fared worse was in the increase in preterm deliveries, a decrease in the mean maternal weight gain during pregnancy, and a decrease in the mean birth weight of the infant. The researchers theorized that the negative consequences were more closely related to IBD disease activity than to the medications taken in an attempt to control the inflammation.

One caution should be noted with the use of sulfasalazine as it competes with folic acid for absorption. Poor folic acid intake has been associated with neural tube birth defects.

For lactation purposes, doctors usually urge their patients to use caution with sulfasalazine or 5-ASA drugs as diarrhea has been reported in some breastfed infants whose mothers were on the medication.

Infliximab (Remicade) is used in the treatment of CD and rheumatoid arthritis. However, very little information exists on the maternal and fetal safety of the medication when used immediately prior to conception or during pregnancy. It is a category B drug.

One small study involving fifty-nine women who used infliximab either at the time of conception or during pregnancy found that the rates of congenital abnormalities and gestational risks were the same as in women who were not exposed to the medication. Animal studies involving the drug would only work in chimpanzees or humans, thus limiting the amount and scope of such studies. The same can be said for nursing information. The company, in prescribing information, states, "It is not known whether Remicade is excreted in human milk or absorbed systemically after ingestion. Because many drugs and immunoglobulins are excreted in human milk, and because of the potential for adverse reactions in nursing infants from Remicade, women should not breast-feed their infants while taking Remicade. A decision should be made whether to discontinue nursing or to discontinue the drug, taking into account the importance of the drug to the mother."

Another category B drug in the biologics is adalimumab (Humira), which is likely to be approved for use in CD in 2007. The drug was tested in gestating monkeys at hundreds of times the human dosage with no ill effects on the mother or fetus. However, there are no studies in pregnant humans at this time, so the makers of the drug suggest using it in women only "if clearly needed." As for lactation, the makers say that it is not known if the drug is excreted in human milk, and the potential for harm to the child may exist. Because of this, the makers say a decision about either discontinuing the drug or discontinuing breast feeding should be made.

The other biologic that is likely to be approved in 2007, certolizumab pegol (Cimzia), is not rated yet, as it has not been approved for other uses as Humira has in the case of rheumatoid arthritis.

Two other medications that are facing the final point of the approval process through the FDA, sargramostim (Leukine) and natalizumab (Tysabri), had both been approved for use in other diseases in the past few years. As a result of animal studies, both are category C drugs. With Tysabri, one study with pregnant female guinea pigs found a small decline in pup survival two weeks after birth, while another study found an increase in miscarriages among pregnant monkeys treated with the drug. The makers of the drug suggest discontinuing the drug if a woman becomes pregnant while on it; they also suggest discontinuing the drug or discontinuing nursing in the case of a lactating woman. No animal studies have been done on the impact of Leukine on the developing fetus, nor is it known if the drug is excreted in breast milk. Because of these facts, the manufacturer says the drug should be used in pregnant or lactating females only "if clearly needed."

Antibiotics such as metronidazole (Flagyl) and ciprofloxacin (Cipro) are also often used in treating IBD as well as other diseases. Studies involving metronidazole suggest that the use of the drug during pregnancy or at the time of conception is not linked with increased congenital abnormalities or gestational risks. Doctors usually limit the use of this category B drug to one to two weeks in duration in the second and third trimester only.

Cipro is a common medication for the treatment of abscesses and infections in CD patients. It is a C category medication, in part because no adequate studies of the effects have been done on humans and few studies have been done in animal models such as rats. In those studies, no maternal or fetal harm was found in the rats. Because such little information exists, doctors usually use the medication only when the benefits outweigh the potential risks and only in short duration such as one to two weeks.

These antibiotics are excreted in the milk of lactating mothers. Because of the potential for adverse reactions in the child, either the drug or nursing should be discontinued.

Rifaximin (Xifaxan) is a newer medication, used by some with CD though not yet specifically approved for that use. Though this drug acts topically to clear undesirable bacteria from the lumen, it has been shown to cause deformations in rats and rabbits, including cleft palate, jaw shortening, and small eyes, when the mother was exposed to the drug at higher levels than that to which humans are exposed. It is not known if the drug is excreted in human milk. The manufacturers suggest that pregnant women be given the drug only when it is needed and that nursing mothers discontinue either the drug or breastfeeding.

Steroids are the next category of drugs of concern for pregnant women with IBD. Experience has shown that drugs such as prednisone or prednisolone have been safe for use during pregnancy for such conditions as asthma, arthritis, and a variety of other conditions, including IBD. Some smaller studies and individual case studies report slightly higher incidence rates of cleft palate and lip in infants born to mothers who took the medication during pregnancy. However, those results were not substantiated in larger studies. Because of this, corticosteroids are in the C class, meaning that there have been possible minimal effects on the fetuses exposed to it in utero.

Budesonide (Entocort) has only been available in the United States since October 2001, but studies conducted in Europe where it has been available for longer suggest that animals receiving the medication had higher amounts of babies born with fetal growth retardation, skeletal delay, and spontaneous abortion. Due to negative results in animal studies, the drug is ranked in category C. However, a study involving data from the Swedish Medical Birth Registry found that no higher amounts of birth defects or pregnancy risks were reported among 2,014 infants whose mothers used Budesonide during pregnancy.

Most doctors say that the use of steroids during lactation is safe, as there has been no significant risk reported with infants of mothers who are on the medications.

With regard to immunosuppressants, cyclosporine is another C class drug that is generally reserved for patients with severe UC. In those cases, the drug in generally used to prevent or delay the occurrence of surgery or in cases where other immunosuppressants are not tolerated. Outside of IBD, the drug is used in the treatment of other autoimmune diseases as well as in post-transplant antirejection therapy.

One Canadian study examined several other studies where the mothers were on cyclosporine at the time of conception or were treated with the drug during pregnancy. Of the 410 cases studied, about half were preterm births. However, there appeared to be no increased risk for congenital malformations in the infants. It is known that the drug can pass from mother to nursing infant. For this reason, it may be wise to avoid breastfeeding while on the drug.

Azathioprine (Azasan and Imuran) and 6-MP have been the subject of a bit of controversy in the past decade regarding the safety of the fetus. Theoretically, the drugs act to slow the production of certain cells. In embryonic and fetal formation, rapid cell division is the key to normal growth.

However, a handful of small studies in women and men who were on the medication for inflammatory bowel disease, other autoimmune diseases such as lupus, and post-transplant immune suppression exist. The findings of those studies include small numbers of abnormalities in the infants born to mothers and fathers taking the medication at the time of conception or during the pregnancy, including one report of multiple digits on the hands or feet (six fingers or six toes) and cleft palate in another. At least three children had blood abnormalities that may be related to the mothers' bone marrow suppression. These findings should be regarded with caution, as the doses of the drugs in some cases were higher than are usually prescribed for

IBD patients, and some of the patients were on other drugs that may have caused the abnormalities. More studies find that the rate of birth defects among children born to women on the medications is closer to four percent, within the normal range of birth defects among all pregnancies. It is important to note that many gastroenterologists do not advise against the use of these drugs during pregnancy.

Still, the medication is in the D class of FDA pregnancy drugs, meaning no obvious risk of congenital malformations exist but some have been reported. Here, the benefit of the drug to the mother to help her carry to term by controlling symptoms is weighed against the potential risk to the fetus. Some doctors suggest that men who are planning to have children with their partner in the near future take a break from immunosuppressive therapy. For lactating mothers, doctors usually warn against using the drug, as it can pass into the breast milk and could cause immunosuppressing in the nursing infant.

Tacrolimus (Prograf) is relatively new in the IBD world of treatment and very few use it at this time. That said, it has plenty of use in the post-transplant world of medicine and has been placed in category C. Over the years since it was introduced, scientists have studied the effect of the drug during pregnancy. In animal models, the drug given in high doses was shown to cause a greater number of stillbirths as well as low birth weight in the live births of rats. It is known that the drug crosses the placenta, and though there are no controlled studies of the drug in pregnant females, some newborns whose mothers took the drug while they were pregnant were found to have higher levels of potassium in their blood or have kidney dysfunction. For this reason, the manufacturers of the drug say that it should be used in pregnant women only when the benefit to the mother outweighs the risk to the fetus. It also warns against nursing while on the drug as the drug is excreted in human milk.

Methotrexate and thalidomide are two drugs that should not be considered in men or women who are planning a pregnancy. Both of these drugs act to suppress certain parts of the immune process and have been beneficial in achieving remission, although thalidomide continues to be tested for its efficacy, and both are used in the treatment of other diseases. However, methotrexate is used in some cases to stimulate an abortion while thalidomide has been positively linked with multiple birth defects. Neither should be used in the mother of a nursing infant, as the immunosuppressive effects can pass into the breast milk. The FDA pregnancy category for these drugs is X.

Childbirth options

In women with IBD, vaginal and C-section births have occurred in a number of situations, from individuals with ostomies to those with minor disease activity, from those with past rectal disease to those with raging ileums. Vaginal birth is not only possible but it happens all the time in both CD and UC patients. However, aside from other complications such as a breech baby or other birth-related complications that necessitate a cesarian section in otherwise healthy women, the major factor in determining if a pregnant woman needs to have a C-section over a vaginal birth specifically with IBD relates to the rigidity of the rectum and the **perineum**. This area moves to accommodate the fetus's head during the process, and a badly scarred perineum and rectum would make that more difficult. Due to this, a C-section is usually recommended ahead of time when rectal disease is present or has caused damage in the area in the past.

IN A SENTENCE:

> *Pregnancy is a common occurrence in IBD patients and may be made safer for the mother and child through careful selection of medication to control symptoms.*

living

Coping with Pregnancy, Childbirth, and Recovery with IBD

FRANKLY PUT, being sick is awful, being sick with a baby is worse, and being sick with a baby and other children is the worst. But sometimes, these scenarios are unavoidable. Coping strategies should be developed.

First of all, it helps to have your obstetrician (OB) and your GI doctor on the same page as far as your treatment is concerned. Discuss the potential for complications with your OB doctor ahead of time and encourage that doctor to discuss your case with your gastroenterologist as well as your colorectal surgeon. Certain plans may have to be made; for example, if your rectum has undergone significant disease activity, the benefits of a C-section birth versus a vaginal birth should be discussed ahead of time.

If you are sick and have to be hospitalized while you are pregnant, the same rules apply for hospitalization in Month 3. If you have small children, have a plan in place ahead of time for who will take care of them when you are not available. The best solution is to have a friend or relative come into your home to care for the children, allowing the little ones the least amount of disruption possible.

Be sure also to maintain adequate nutrition and hydration during pregnancy. This may be difficult when you are laid up with morning sickness as well as disease symptoms. Eating small but frequent meals and sipping on electrolyte beverages can help make this an attainable goal.

If the birth will be a C-section, be sure to discuss this with your colorectal surgeon ahead of time. While the abdominal cavity is open for the birth, the surgeon may want to also perform strictureplasty or even resection in certain areas. This two-for-one approach may save you from additional surgery down the line and overlap the recovery for both procedures.

Following the birth, you can make your life easier through a few simple changes:

○ Don't be a hero. Doing it all yourself is not even a good idea when you are well. However, wearing yourself down by taking on the task of caring for a newborn while sick is much worse. Ask for help from the baby's father, your parents, his parents, other relatives, neighbors, friends, and acquaintances. If you have the means to do so, hire a nurse for the first month.

○ Plan ahead. You know you are going to have a baby far before you hit the labor and delivery room. Line up all that help from the people in the previous tip before Junior makes his debut. Fill your freezer with fully prepared meals that can be thawed, reheated, and served at a moment's notice. Stock up your pantry with staples to reduce trips to the outside world in those first few weeks.

○ Don't be afraid to bottle feed. According to pediatricians, the best food for a child is breast milk. Some say that a tighter maternal-infant bond with the child results from breastfeeding, that the child gains a few IQ points as well, and that there is less colic in breastfed babies. The pressure is clearly on. But if you are on a medication that can harm the child, the bottle is probably best. If you are recovering from childbirth and dealing with disease symptoms, a bottle may be the only way to go. Trust me, the child will be fine. All seven of the children in my family were bottle fed, we are extremely close with my mother, and five of the seven had merit-based scholarships to college. Besides, my son was breastfed and he had colic for four and a half very long months.

○ If you do breastfeed, hydration is even more crucial, as the process itself causes the loss of fluids. Having diarrhea makes this worse. While feeding the child, grab a glass of water or an electrolyte-containing beverage to stave off dehydration.

○ Rest. A rested body is well on the way to recovery and is better able to withstand the stress of parenthood.

When your child is old enough for outings, there are a few things you can do to make this easier as well. For one, bathroom stops are inevitable but may pose a problem with a stroller. In instances where a trusted friend or relative is not available to watch the child, use the handicap stall and take the stroller in with you. Also, when packing the diaper and bottle bag, save room for a drink for yourself. Joining a class or playgroup with other mothers may also help you to realize that the struggles you may associate with being a parent with IBD are really the same struggles that all new parents face.

Above all, be sure to enjoy this time. You will never have these days back. Though at times you might be grateful for this, it really is a time to savor.

IN A SENTENCE:

> *Managing the end of the pregnancy and the first few weeks of a child's life can be done with the help of others.*

Living
Daily Life

IN THE days following your diagnosis, leaving your home may have been nearly unthinkable; even now, eight months after the diagnosis, the symptoms may not have reached their zenith. That is because your home is likely safe and secure from some of the uncertainties these diseases force upon the human soul. In your home, you likely always have access to a clean and comfortable bathroom where you could let loose without a care. Your refrigerator and pantry offer a variety of safe and healthy food choices. There is little risk in obtaining a cold or other communicable illness if you are on immunosuppressant medication and you stay home all the time. It is a controlled environment in almost every respect.

But you can't live in a bubble. At some point, you have to leave that secure environment and rejoin the rest of the world as you pursue a life once again. The first thing you must do on your return to a normal lifestyle is to relearn how to navigate the pitfalls—or rather pit stops—of daily life. And the sooner you do that, the better.

Everyday living

For practical purposes, you can't really tote around a portable toilet, so learning how to handle urgent needs in public will take you far. The first line of defense can be medicine. Antidiarrheal or antispasmodic agents, if safe to use, can make the occurrence of diarrhea less frequent and more manageable. Stool bulking agents are also helpful for some.

When these are not possible or don't work as well, the next helpful thing to know is the location of all bathrooms—public and private. When in a public location such as a shopping mall or theater, bathrooms are usually located not far from the entrances or in an alcove. In restaurants or grocery stores, they are usually located near the entrance or somewhere near a food preparation area, as it is easiest to install plumbing for the different facilities in the same wall. In any case, it helps to ask someone for directions to the bathroom immediately upon entering such a place, if for no other reason than peace of mind.

Not all bathrooms are public, however. The vast majority of workplaces have private facilities out of range of the public. For example, within a store of the mall, you may feel the sudden, strong urge to go to the bathroom, yet you are a full 100 yards from the nearest public facility. Not every vendor will let individuals use these private facilities. In such cases, it helps to carry with you a special card issued by the Crohn's & Colitis Foundation of America. The card, issued with membership, in bold lettering states, "I can't wait. Thank you for understanding. The bearer of this card has a medical condition that requires him/her to use the bathroom facilities urgently. Thank you for your cooperation." Present the card to the storeowner, apologize for any inconvenience, quickly explain that you desperately need to use their bathroom, and ask to use the facilities. Even the staunchest storeowner or manager may let you behind the counter once they know it is a medical emergency, not just the case of someone who is too lazy to walk the distance to the public facilities. Be sure to thank them profusely afterward.

When you are on the road and feel the urge to use the bathroom, the best places to stop are fast food restaurants. For one, they are open most hours of the day and night. For another, they are generally accepting of individuals who come in to use the facilities. If you have the cash on hand, buy lemonade or hot tea on your way out to show your appreciation.

Sometimes, an accident can happen, especially if fecal incontinence has become an issue. If this is the case, handle it as quickly as possible. Some people do this by carrying a change of clothing in their cars at all times; others keep a change of underwear in a plastic bag in their purses or backpacks. Don't feel bad. Realize that these things happen, then clean up and move on.

Picnics, entertainment, and other social occasions

With the advent of cable, high definition television, and other home theater accessories, there have been fewer reasons to leave the home. But not all events are televised, nor should you become a hermit.

When purchasing tickets to a planned activity such as a concert, a ball game, or a theater performance, try to get tickets on the aisle. This way you are able to leave your seat with the least amount of disruptions when the need arises. Before you leave for the event, it can be very helpful to call the venue ahead of time to make arrangements for special bathroom privileges as toilet facilities can become quite congested during such events and may be located in inconvenient areas. By calling ahead and explaining your special circumstances, you may request to use the bathroom facilities normally relegated to workers or ask if there are less congested options. I have done this on several occasions. Often, I am told to introduce myself to one of the managers who is briefed on my need. I have been escorted down some darkened halls but it is worth it to not have to wait in a long line.

For outdoor activities such as picnics, calling the organizers ahead of time and explaining your need of bathroom facilities can alleviate some fears. For these events and other occasions such as weddings or similar celebrations, take the time to ask about the menu as well. Sometimes, alterations or special requests can be made if you bring them to the host's attention ahead of time. If there is little that you can eat that will be served, be sure to eat before you arrive.

Eating out

With a special diet, it may seem that the only things you can eat are those you prepare yourself, seemingly leaving you little option but to cower in your kitchen and turn down all social invitations. With a little planning and creativity, however, you can safely enjoy a meal at just about any restaurant.

When you enter a restaurant, be sure to first check out the bathrooms. This is important not only to wash your hands before you eat, but also to know the location of the bathroom stalls in case the need should arise during the meal. Another big benefit of visiting the restrooms is to check out the cleanliness of the facilities. In general, restaurant managers are as fastidious about the cleanliness of the bathrooms as they are about the cleanliness of their kitchen. If the garbage is overflowing, the sinks are gooey with spilled soap, or the toilets are in need of a scrub, the kitchen is probably not much better, leaving the door open for bacterial, food-borne illnesses such as campylobacter, hepatitis A and E. coli—all dangerous illnesses to the general public, but especially to those who are immune-suppressed or have digestive illnesses. Leave the restaurant if the bathroom is not up to inspection.

When you sit down to eat, check out the menus. Look for foods that are steamed, baked, or broiled, and skip over the selections that are covered with cheese, in fatty sauces, sautéd, or fried. One great clue to such entrees on a menu is if they are accompanied by a "heart healthy" symbol. Be aware of any other food restrictions or sensitivities you might have at the time. Ask the wait staff about how the food is prepared or what special ingredients are used; for example, marinated meats are often soaked in oil, thus upping their fat content. Cooks and chefs receive requests for special diets on a regular basis and are usually happy to accommodate any requests such as eliminating cheese, putting a sauce on the side, or steaming all vegetables to oblivion. If you are unsure about a certain item or what can be ordered, explain your restrictions and ask the chef for suggestions. Also, if your selection doesn't turn out the way you envisioned, don't be afraid to send it back. It happens all the time.

While it may seem that you can't eat at a fast food restaurant due to the usually fatty and salty meals served in such establishments, let me assure you that it is possible, given extra vigilance. And this fact is really important to know since the average American eats more than four meals away from home each week and half of all American adults are restaurant patrons each day, according to the National Restaurant Association. With fast food restaurants making up the bulk of all restaurants, never eating at one may be near impossible.

Because most of us dine in such facilities at one time or another, it might be helpful to learn about the best choices before entering the doors. All of the major fast food restaurants—McDonald's, Wendy's, Burger King, Arby's, etc.—maintain websites, on which they carry nutritional information about each of their menu selections. Here, you can find out which entrée has the least amount of fat, where baked potatoes can be had, if a pasta and salad bar is available, which salad dressings are low-fat or fat free. As an example, you may learn that the seemingly innocuous breakfast menu item contains 30 grams of fat and one gram of salt while the muffin has considerably less of both. Baked chicken sandwiches are usually the best selections, made even better by skipping any bacon, cheese, or mayonnaise. Lemonade and fruit punches are available and may be better selections than pop. You get the picture. I find that the best places to eat are usually bagel shops. Nearly all of the selections are low in fat, and lactose-free spreads such as hummus or jelly are usually available.

Also, ethnic restaurants have been enjoying an increase in popularity over the past two decades. It is a good thing, too, because many have abundantly flavorful selections that are low in fat, baked, steamed, or served with a side of rice or bread. Again, watch out for the key trouble words such as "fried" and order all of your vegetables fork tender if stricturing is a problem.

On the rare occasion when you are roped into going to a restaurant where you see no good food choices on the horizon, eat beforehand, if possible, or pick at the bread basket.

Exercising

If staying active when you are healthy is a challenge, staying active when your disease is in full force may seem like an insurmountable task. But exercise is an important part of life, something that no one should live without. Studies show that regular exercise improves heart and lung function, stimulates brain activity, increases bone density, lubricates the joints, tones the muscles, staves off serious conditions such as obesity, cardiovascular diseases, and certain cancers, and contributes to a sense of well-being.

However, the effects of IBD can keep even the fittest of individuals away from the gym for weeks at a stretch and can make others forfeit their routines entirely. Fevers suck the energy from anyone, as can anemia. Feeling the urge to use the bathroom can prevent people from starting that five-mile jog. Steroids like prednisone can weaken the long muscles in the body, making any thigh work exponentially more difficult. Simply moving around more can cause greater peristalsis, leading to more bathroom trips.

Because of this, getting started on or continuing an exercise program when you are ill can be difficult but is possible by making some modifications to your routine.

- ○ If you do high-impact aerobic exercise, you may find that you have to leave the floor often to use the bathroom. Switching to a less jarring, lower-impact or water-based version of the same exercise will provide the same cardiovascular benefits while being gentler on the body.
- ○ Running or walking outdoors can be peaceful and relaxing but it can also cause anxiety if the act of doing so stimulates the bowel function in the absence of a toilet. Finding an outside track or a state park with open bathroom facilities and plotting a course where you can still be in easy reach of the toilet can allow you to continue your routine. Also, taking an antidiarrheal drug prior to stretching can also help to slow the GI tract.
- ○ While taking immunosuppressive medication, going to a public or private gym can be an invitation to illness, as gym equipment and bathroom facilities can harbor a ton of illness-causing germs. People who work out think nothing of wiping their sweaty upper lips and then grasping weights or equipment, facilitating that germ transfer to you. Or how about those who prefer to sit naked on the benches in the locker room? Short of sanitizing each piece of equipment before you use it, scrupulous handwashing is your only defense. My personal solution to this (after several consecutive illnesses derived from the gym) was to quit the gym and use the annual fee to purchase a new piece of equipment for my home every year. The result is a professional gym in my basement, steps from my bathroom, no waiting in lines to use equipment or weights, and total control of the television content. If you can't get away from working out in a gym, try to exercise during times when gym traffic is at its lowest.
- ○ Check out yoga and tai chi classes. These are gentle yet effective ways to up your exercise volume and are usually held in studios

close to a bathroom. Before signing up for a formal class in an expensive studio, try out the method at your local YMCA or city-sponsored parks and recreation division to see if you like it.

○ Weight training strengthens not only muscles but bones as well. With minimal investment, it can be done in the home. Before investing in a set of weights, however, it might be prudent to hire a personal trainer for a few sessions to learn the proper techniques.

○ Exercise videos are a great way of working out for people with IBD. They are relatively cheap, require little to no extra equipment, and are used in the home at your convenience, making bathroom accessibility a moot point. Before investing in the tape, you can rent them from the library or from most video outlets to see if you like the content.

○ For anyone into hiking or other rigorous outdoor activities, bathrooms become a luxury, not a necessity. In these instances, be sure to relieve your bowels away from natural water sources. If possible, dig a small hole in which to go to the bathroom, use toilet paper to wipe, and fill in the hole. Bring along antibacterial wipes for cleaning your hands when you are through.

○ Because you have IBD, your risk of dehydration can be higher during flare-ups. With this in mind, be sure to remain hydrated while working out by increasing consumption of water and electrolytes.

Be aware that there are definitely times when you need to avoid working out or cut back on the intensity of the workout. Fever is an indication that workouts should be ceased for the time as not heeding these symptoms can lead to greater dehydration or heat stroke. Stop working out if your symptoms include dizziness or nausea or if you notice an increase in symptoms. When the symptoms have abated, begin working out again but shorten the exercise time and decrease the intensity of the workouts for a few days or weeks until your strength returns.

Getting dressed

With IBD symptoms present, you may find that the snug but comfortable jeans you adore are cutting you in two. Or perhaps that favorite pair of loafers are practically splitting at the seams during a bout of arthritis.

Making bathroom access the law

Since you are already in the eighth month post-diagnosis, you may already know that no matter how nicely you ask or how urgent and evident your need is, some shopkeepers are still going to turn down your request to use the bathroom.

I know this personally because it has happened to me more often than not. After one particular incident in a Kids' Foot Locker, I decided to complain to a government body because I felt my rights had been violated. There have been public concessions for people with other disabilities for years. Handicap parking spaces and ramps, special phones for the deaf, Braille menus for the blind all exist to help people with other disabilities, I reasoned. So bathroom access for those of us who face that challenge should governed as well, right?

It turns out that it isn't. And the only way to change this situation, the government lawyer explained to me, was to create such a law. So, in 2000, I met with my state representative, Andy Meisner, and educated him regarding the importance of this issue. Working together, we developed a bill that would provide greater access to private "employee-only" bathrooms in businesses that are open to the public. In businesses where there are two or more employees, access to that bathroom must be granted to individuals who present a doctor's note explaining the need for the bathroom due to the individual's medical condition that causes either fecal or urinary incontinence. The bill states that if the business refuses this access, it can face a fine of up to $100.

While the bill has been reintroduced in Michigan and remains in the Commerce Committee, other states have followed Michigan's lead. In Illinois, a national CCFA board member heard about our actions and put an Illinois state legislator's office in contact with me. They copied the legislation I provided and introduced it. After passing the house and senate, it was signed into law by the governor of that state. Legislators in Texas, Ohio, and Minnesota are planning to introduce the same legislation in 2007, and activists in Maryland are hoping to amend that state's law to reflect the provisions in Michigan's bill.

It would be great if all business owners understood the plight of those who have IBD, especially the fear of not having access to a bathroom in public. But that doesn't always happen. Until that situation changes, it might be wise to introduce this legislation in all fifty states. If you are interested in doing so in your own state, please feel free to contact me through the RevolutionHealth.com Web site listed in the resources section or through the Michigan chapter of the CCFA at Michigan@ccfa.org.

Whatever the case, you aren't comfortable in your body and your body sure isn't comfortable in its clothes.

During these times, it helps to choose clothing that is more forgiving. For example, women who feel bloated after eating or due to symptoms may find that pregnancy pantyhose offer an elegant look without squeezing the gut. Elasticized or drawstring pants work in less formal situations rather than belts; these are also easier to dispense with during a dash to the toilet. Support hose or socks purchased from a medical supply shop can help reduce swelling in the lower joints while providing a comfortable "hug" to the affected joints. Trade the shoes as soon as you are home for a comforting pair of slippers.

IN A SENTENCE:

> *Make adjustments to your daily routine so you can continue to enjoy life.*

learning

Remission:
Life Beyond Disease

REMISSION IS a wonderful state of being, a veritable vacation from misery. Symptoms decrease in severity or disappear entirely, appetite returns, food choices multiply, and less medicine is needed. Life returns to normal, or at least a semblance of normal.

Defining remission

Doctors have struggled for decades to define exactly when a patient had active disease and when remission was achieved. In both CD and UC, the result was a series of medical algorithms that purport to measure disease activity or the lessening of such by assigning points and grades to both perceived and actual changes. Usually, the higher the number or lower the grade, the greater disease activity there is; conversely, the lower the number and higher the grade, the less disease activity there is.

In CD, the most common such scale is called the Crohn's Disease Activity Index (CDAI). It takes the accumulation of daily measures for one week of the number of soft or liquid stools a patient has, the degree of abdominal pain (rated 0 for none to 3 for severe), and the person's general well-being (rated 0 for well to 4 for terrible). This score is added to ratings of other factors such as the number of current extraintestinal manifestations, whether or not the patient is using an antidiarrheal medication, abdominal pain measurement while taking into account a rise or fall in hemocrit, and body weight. If the score is greater than 150, the patient is considered to have active disease. If the score is lower than 150, the patient is considered to be in remission.

Other algorithms take into account pediatric symptoms, anal symptoms, endoscopic indications, and inflammatory symptoms. Generally, however, a doctor can surmise a patient's condition by taking into account their symptoms as well as their reliance on and use of certain medications.

For UC, the algorithms rely upon that which is seen via endoscope and examined through biopsies. They look for microscopic changes and also take into account the possibility for colorectal cancer development. These results are used often for the description of symptoms of research subjects, not in daily practice. Again, doctors generally rely on the patient's report of symptoms and their reliance on and use of certain medications.

What remission feels like

Remission usually doesn't happen in the time frame in which a patient expects it. When symptoms are bad, most patients wouldn't mind if remission entered their life in the next day, if not the next minute. However, it can take months to years of medical and surgical treatment before remission is achieved.

But when it does happen, it is a beautiful thing. In fact, it may leave the patient wondering how they endured their time of abdominal pain, fevers, and unpredictable bowel movements.

Of course, the definition of remission will vary from person to person. For those whose first experience with mild to moderate symptoms wanes, the frequency and consistency of bowel movements will become more predictable and normal. For those who have had resections or have extensive scarring, it can mean that the new normal is merely the lessening of pain and the absence of extraintestinal manifestations as diarrhea continues due to the physiological alteration of bowel function. For those with ostomies due to UC, remission may be permanent if the entire colon and rectum is removed. For those with ostomies due to CD, the disease can return.

Remission does not equal cure

It may be tempting to those who attain remission to pour the pills down the drain or lose their doctor's number. After all, with no or few symptoms to speak of, it is hard to justify maintaining the routines established during times of illness. But CD and UC are chronic conditions, meaning they can return time and time again.

However, there are a few things that patients might want to consider to maintain and prolong their remission. The first thing they can do is to continue taking maintenance medication if it is prescribed to them. Immunosuppressives are commonly taken for years when no symptoms are present as the continued suppression of the immune system keeps the diseases from returning. Sulfasalazine and the 5-ASA drugs Pentasa, Dipentum, Rowasa, and Asacol have both been indicated positively in studies as helping to sustain remission in UC patients and CD patients with ileal, colonic, or rectal disease. A minority of doctors prescribe low-dose prednisone over the long haul to small numbers of patients to achieve and maintain remission; that said, other doctors don't believe remission can be attained until the patient is free and clear of steroids. One exception is budesonide (Entocort); that drug appears to help maintain remission in CD patients with ileal and right-sided colonic disease at a maintenance dose of 6 mg daily.

Since it was the first of the biologic medications to be approved for CD, infliximab (Remicade) has been used as a maintenance medication, with patients who use the drug submitting to infusions once every five to eight weeks. The other biologic drugs that are likely to be approved shortly, adalimumab (Humira) and certolizumab (Cimzia), will most likely also have a regular dosing regimen for remission maintenance. Antiobiotics like metronidazole (Flagyl) and ciprofloxacin (Cipro) are both used in maintenance doses in people who have issues with perianal disease or who struggle with recurring abscesses and resulting fistulas.

Maintaining a relationship with your doctor should also be a priority. Although you may attend one or two appointments annually, it is still important to keep the lines of communication open to report the reappearance of symptoms and to obtain medication refills. For those with increased colon cancer risk, it is vital to maintain contact for annual or regular colonoscopies. In particular, a patient can also use the time with the doctor for the administration of a flu shot. For these reasons, it might be helpful to schedule one appointment in the spring for the colonoscopy and one prior to flu season for the flu shot.

A continued awareness of early symptoms can prevent an exacerbation from becoming a full-blown relapse in some individuals. By reporting the symptoms as soon as they appear, milder medications can be used to rein them in. That doesn't mean that the symptoms won't escalate or stronger medications won't be used, but for damage control purposes, it is best to catch the symptoms early on.

IN A SENTENCE:

> *While remission is a wonderful change of pace for those who have been ill for a while, it requires that patients remain vigilant over their care.*

living

Travel
and IBD

THERE IS nothing quite as relaxing as a vacation, a chance to enjoy a week or more away from the daily grind. And everyone needs one. Research shows that workers who take regular vacations are more productive, more relaxed, and happier than their counterparts who do not take advantage of a break.

But getting away from a routine in the comfort of predictable surroundings can be nerve-wracking for those with IBD. Questions about healthy food choices and the accessibility of toilets are overshadowed only by the fear of becoming ill while away from home. However, with a little extra planning, vacations are manageable ways to kick back and take your mind off your illness while you recharge your energy.

Get packing

Because a trip starts long before you board the plane or train or put the keys in the ignition, you will probably be thinking about what you will be bringing with you. You may plan your outfits, laying them out on the bed before packing. Many people pack extra socks and underwear, adding some to both checked baggage and carry-ons. If you are like me, you also backtrack over what you use in the morning—blow-dryer, brush, toothbrush, toothpaste, makeup, deodorant, perfume, robe, and slippers—and gather it all to go into the luggage. And, of course, in this ever-changing world marked by terrorism, you should always check with the Transportation Security Administration (tsa.gov) for any restrictions on the content of suitcases.

At this time, it is a good idea to also gather the items you use in the treatment of your disease. Medications—prescription and over the counter—should be packed in their original bottles. I carry twice the amount I will need in two sets of bottles, in two separate bags, one to check and one to carry on board. This way, if one of the bags is missing, lost or stolen, I at least have one set of medication to use. Some people also carry an extra set of prescriptions with them for the same reason; although a doctor's prescription may not be honored in another state or country, another physician will be able to see what your physician ordered and issue a more valid prescription.

For individuals with ostomies, extra supplies such as appliances, adhesives, and plastic bags in which to dispose of the used supplies should be added to both bags. For those using anal dilators, packing them in a plastic bag with a doctor's prescription describing its use has helped me get through many airport screenings.

If you are traveling by train or plane, it is also helpful to pack a few food items and bottled water to tide you over until you reach your destination. Although airlines and train companies can reserve a special meal for you, don't count on it actually making the destination. For this reason, a bagel, bananas, pretzels, Rice Krispie Treats, cereal bars, baked potato chips, bottled water, and juice boxes packed into carry-on luggage can help to sustain you during the travel time. Again, be sure to log on to tsa.gov for the latest restrictions regarding luggage contents.

For car trips, the same principle applies. A small cooler or ice chest can be packed with safe foods such as sandwiches and snacks that can be consumed at a roadside park equipped with a bathroom. This is really a healthier option for all in the car, as some choices from fast food restaurants can pack on the pounds through excessive fat and calories.

Another helpful item to pack is hand sanitizer, a liquid soap that needs no water for washing. This is especially true for those on immunosuppressive medication. Often, bathrooms in train depots, airline terminals, or state parks are not the cleanest of facilities, at times bereft of soap and paper towels. A dab of hand sanitizer can help to kill any illness-causing germs that can easily spoil a vacation.

Karen unfortunately learned this lesson the hard way with her daughter Kate, a CD patient. While on a trip, a stomach bug invaded the family, sending Kate to the hospital. "So now, I make sure everyone in the family uses hand sanitizer after they touch anything and before they eat, if handwashing is not a possibility. I admit to being a full-fledged germ freak while traveling, but we have been lucky enough to have had a number of healthy trips in a row, so I think it is paying off," she said.

Planes, trains, and automobiles

Now that you are packed and prepared, it is time to face the next hurdle: travel. The amount of planning is reflective on the severity of the disease at the time of your departure. If you are in remission or are experiencing mild symptoms, you may not need to make any changes in your routine whatsoever. However, if your disease is more active, you may want to follow some of these suggestions.

For car travel, the greatest part of the planning comes in plotting your course for restrooms and meal breaks. The goal here is to make the unpredictable and unknown predictable and known. For this exercise, it is helpful to have a map of the area to which you are traveling, a travel guide from the state or states through which you will pass, and the Internet. On the map, plot your course and then mark off the major cities where you know facilities will be available. Using the travel guide and an Internet map service such as www.mapquest.com, locate areas such as parks or rest stops for picnic or bathroom stops; state police posts also have access to that information. In areas where stretches of road appear desolate, use the websites of major fast food and family restaurants to try to locate a facility along the route.

Emily finds these places to be the best for quick bathroom stops. "If I'm in a car I schedule regular stops even if I don't feel like I have to go to the bathroom right then," she said. "Also, if I'm sightseeing in a new city and can't find a public bathroom I pop into a department store or a hotel lobby."

While driving, be on the lookout for signs of restaurants of any kind. Where food is served, a bathroom will be close at hand. When all else fails, nature it. By that I mean pull over and head for the closest, most private area to relieve yourself. If bears and foxes do it, you can, too. At least one individual I know improvises a bathroom by pulling over to the side of the road, opening both passenger side doors, stretching a towel behind her to seal off the car, and using the door frame as a brace to steady herself as she goes. It seems a bit acrobatic for my tastes, but it has worked for her in the past when she had no other options.

Airplane trips and short train rides pose their own dilemmas with food and bathrooms. Bathroom facilities in both are usually small, cramped, foul smelling, and shared by around a hundred other individuals. They are entirely inaccessible during the time when the vehicles begin to move or when they are in the process of stopping. Because of this, bathroom accessibility or lack thereof can be anxiety-provoking.

To remedy this, you may want to consider forgoing food prior to traveling and consuming only water until you reach your destination. With fewer physical prompts for peristalsis, there may be less need to use the bathroom.

Another prudent step to take in securing bathroom access is to tell the attendant upon boarding of your condition and your reliance on swift bathroom access. If you are in coach seating, ask if you can use the first class facilities if the need arises. Using this approach on dozens of trips with different carriers, I have yet to be turned down; on the contrary, the attendants were often sympathetic and checked on me during the flight to make sure I was okay.

Lynn, a seasoned traveler with IBD, employs a different method to confront the issue of inadequate bathroom access. "When I travel, I usually wear a Depend undergarment and carry an extra in my carry-on bag," she said, adding that she may not soil the adult diaper but the security of knowing it is okay to do so is a comfort.

Most airlines do not offer food service, providing instead an array of low-fat snacks for sale and allowing travelers to bring on board other food items for consumption. Some airlines offer limited food service in first class, including a low-fat plate. Amtrak offers a wide selection of hot entrées and cold sandwiches that fit the needs of many with special requests. However, don't count on these foods to be available to you during your travel time. By following the packing rule for safe travel treats, you will avoid this problem.

If you take the train on overnight trips, it is worth it to pay the extra amount for a sleeping room with a private bathroom available in the room.

Be sure to bring along room freshener as some of the facilities are separated from the beds by little more than a stiff curtain.

Bathroom accessibility is often not an issue when traveling on a cruise ship, as staterooms often boast individual bathroom facilities. Where you do have to exercise some caution is in the cleanliness of the kitchen facilities, something over which you have no control and may be completely dependent upon. Bad health reports from the kitchen and dining room can make for an increase in germ-borne stomach illnesses. Cruise line reputations on this issue range from sloppy to sterling. The U.S. government monitors the conditions regularly through surprise health inspections. To find out how your cruise ship fared before you board, you can check out its latest inspection through the Centers for Disease Control's Vessel Sanitation Program at www.cdc.gov.

Foreign travel

Foreign travel is always an issue for individuals with IBD. On the bathroom accessibility issue, it may be helpful to learn the native language phrases for "Where is the bathroom?" as well as the customs regarding use of paper in the facilities. In developing countries, it is not a bad idea to bring your own toilet paper, as the selections there are rougher than the cushiony soft American variety.

Of greater concern is the chance of contracting a gastrointestinal illness from the local water supply or from lessened water and food sanitation levels. Before you find your passport, find out what food- or water-borne illnesses are of a concern using the CDC's Web site. Once in the country, drink only bottled water without ice. Avoid raw fruits and vegetables, unless you have peeled them and not rinsed them with local water. Avoid shellfish, as an increased hepatitis risk is associated with it in certain countries. Avoid any food made by street vendors. For more tips, see the CDC's Web site.

The same rules apply to bringing your own prepared food and snacks when you are unsure of what foods will be available. Any prepackaged foods such as tins of tuna, fruit cups, cereal bars, juice boxes, crackers, peanut butter, jelly, and cereal can be easily packed in baggage to be checked; encase the goods in double plastic bags to seal in any spills. I know it can be a hassle but it can save you from starving when no good food is available.

Should you become ill while you are abroad, finding good health care may be an issue. It might be wise to contact the American embassy in the country of choice prior to traveling to find out what health care options exist should an emergency arise. Some gastroenterologists have colleagues in other countries to whom they can refer you in case of an overseas health crisis. For this reason, ask your GI for a letter of referral to carry with you while you are abroad. It may also help to know the foreign equivalents or translated names of the medications you take. The CCFA carries such a list on its Web site (www.ccfa.org).

IN A SENTENCE:

> *With a few precautions and preparations, you can travel even if you have IBD.*

learning

Insurance and IBD

THERE IS no better argument for the importance of health insurance with IBD than when the actual bill for the first surgery arrives—a heart-attack-provoking $30,000 or more—and the bottom line shows that the insured person has to pay the equivalent of a car payment, with the rest being covered by insurance. Other kinds of insurance such as life insurance and long-term disability insurance are equally important to those with chronic illnesses. And I'll bet you have felt this rather acutely in the past nine months.

That said, these kinds of insurance can be difficult matters for many IBD patients. The dizzying array of options—HMOs, PPOs, traditional coverage—and varied price scales easily push some individuals to select their coverage blindly and hope for the best. Worse, rejections for coverage often send some in a mad attempt to be covered by anything available, leading to less than great coverage. Because of these possibilities, education about available options and rights afforded by law can go a long way.

Health insurance

When starting a new job in a company of some size, one of the first people likely to knock on your cubicle separator or office door will be a benefits coordinator or human resources worker who handles such matters. And in their hands will be a stack of papers you will need to sign to obtain insurance coverage, health insurance being one of the options. Consider this your first homework assignment.

Many companies offer a few plans for coverage, varying from health maintenance organizations (HMOs) to preferred provider organizations (PPOs) to the more traditional, fee-for-service insurance, and other variations. Some companies cover the total cost of the insurance while others will require a deduction from the regular paycheck to pay for a portion of the insurance bill. With the latter case, in general, the more comprehensive the coverage, the larger the deduction.

Understanding the choices is half the battle. Generally, an HMO provides a slew of services such as doctor visits for annual and emergent needs, surgical care, hospital stays, emergency room visits, and tests. Usually, one doctor, called a primary care physician (PCP), coordinates all care and is the one who makes referrals to specialists. In return for the care provided, the subscriber pays a timely fee and/or a small copay like ten dollars for a doctor visit. Doctors who participate in HMOs agree to receive a schedule of fees per patient.

The catch here is that not all doctors take HMO coverage for a variety of reasons, and those who do can terminate their contracts at certain times, forcing the patient to find an HMO-affiliated health care provider. Also, the HMO may limit treatment to what it sees as more common practice. The result is that the patient has fewer choices in doctors to see and fewer hospitals to visit for treatment; the cost of the treatment by nonsubscribing health care providers and hospitals may not be covered, with the cost going to the patient. Additionally, certain treatments may not be covered, leaving the patient to pay the full out of pocket cost.

With PPOs, many services like emergent and preventative care that the HMOs cover are similarly covered. Additionally, participating health care providers and institutions like hospitals are used and often referred to as a "network." Visits to other "out-of-network" health care providers and institutions are partially covered, with the excess cost assigned to the patient.

One way they differ is that the PPO requires that an annual deductible of a set amount (from two hundred to two thousand dollars or more) be paid before coverage kicks in. Even when the coverage does begin, a small copay for services is usually required, the amount or percentage of which varies from service to service and plan to plan.

Traditional fee-for-service coverage is the type of insurance most people had before the creation of PPOs and HMOs. In this coverage, individuals pay a monthly amount, called a premium, as well as an annual deductible in exchange for services. Usually, the patient pays a percentage of the cost of services provided until a certain amount of out of pocket fees have been covered, called a cap. When the cap has been met, the insurance covers all expenses. The coverage is often divided into basic (covering preventative care, some hospitalization, and surgery) and major medical (covering expensive, long-term care for illnesses and injuries); these can be purchased separately in some cases, but many insurance companies combine the two.

While traditional coverage is generally the most expensive option, it allows for greater freedom in choosing doctors and hospitals for coverage. Still, limits are placed on how much of a service or a fee the company will fund, leaving the patient to pay the rest of the bill.

Prescription coverage varies from plan to plan, regardless of the type of insurance offered. Some plans offer no prescription coverage, while others will cover any medication with a ten- to twenty-dollar copay per prescription.

The type of insurance that is best for you depends on the individual situation. For example, if a CD patient's surgeon, gastroenterologist, primary care physician, and hospital are a part of the network and the patient's funds are limited, a PPO may be the best choice. However, if that PPO does not cover medication, that same patient may find that the more expensive traditional plan is a better buy since monthly prescriptions for IBD drugs can reach into the thousands of dollars. Other lifestyle factors such as preventative care coverage for children or location of the closest providers will also factor into a decision.

For those who are independent contractors or employed in a small company that does not offer health insurance benefits, finding health care insurance can involve a bit more work but is still possible. Trade associations (for example, the state's bar association if the patient is a lawyer) often offer health insurance at group or individual rates. Often, the association offers fewer choices than a large company would, but it is better than nothing. City or area chambers of commerce also frequently offer insurance to individuals who own a business within its jurisdiction. Again, choices may be limited.

Another option some insurance companies offer is open enrollment for individuals. With one or two enrollment periods within a year, the companies offer a variety of plan structures. Be warned that individual plans are more expensive than the individual rates are within a group plan.

Long-term disability insurance

Another type of insurance that some individuals with CD or UC may want to investigate is long-term disability insurance. This type of insurance will provide income to the patient should they become disabled due to the course of their disease or as a result of some other catastrophic incident.

What the coverage is depends upon the insurance contract and the situation that befalls the individual. Some will cover only half of the income for the individual and only for a set amount of time. Other plans only supplement that which is paid by Social Security disability. Often, there is a waiting period before the benefits kick in; for example, an individual who is injured or sick and can't work will begin to receive benefits ninety days after the work ends.

There are a few drawbacks to this type of insurance. First, not all companies offer this option to their employees. Second, individual coverage can be very expensive to maintain as it is often based on the person's income. Third, some provisions limit coverage to those who cannot perform absolutely any aspect of their job, meaning that if they can work in some capacity or in a related job, they will not receive benefits. Fourth, insurance companies often require a visit to one of their own doctors, an individual who may not be willing to declare disability. Fifth, the insurance companies often fight the claims, leading to a long legal battle that can deplete a portion of the benefits.

Life insurance

Because better management techniques and treatments are now available for IBD patients, fewer and fewer individuals will die of the diseases or related complications, thus making IBD patients' life expectancy the same as the healthy population. Still, it may be difficult for IBD patients to obtain life insurance policies. It's not personal; in fact, life insurance companies refuse individuals with all sorts of physical and mental illnesses, as well as those with bad habits such as an addiction to cigarettes.

Generally, the best bet with life insurance is to go with a plan that companies often offer their employees. You probably won't get a million dollar policy, but you may have the option to increase or decrease the benefit amount. Sometimes, this insurance can be continued as an individual policy after employment terminates.

If you have to purchase the insurance independently, there are generally two kinds of insurance available for purchase. The first and least expensive is term insurance. For a set amount of time, the individual is covered under certain conditions. The younger the person, the cheaper the insurance. The second kind is whole life insurance. This option allows a person to pay a monthly premium that accumulates through investment. During the life of the individual the money can be borrowed and is usually released to the individual at a predetermined time.

In either case, the amount of the payment may be higher for those with chronic illness as the risk of death, however small it may be, is already present. Also, it is wise to be aware of all of the loopholes that let the insurance company off the hook in certain death situations. For example, an accidental death policy only covers death as the result of certain accidental situations, not illness-related causes.

Insurance for children with IBD

For the most part, children with IBD can expect the same protection their parents or guardians enjoy under COBRA and HIPAA, two laws explained on the next page. They are also usually covered under their parents' medical plans at least until age eighteen. In most plans, coverage can be extended through college and possibly graduate school as long as the student maintains a minimum number of credit hours per semester. The young adults can either find a job where insurance benefits can then take over, or can scout out their own insurance.

If you think you can't afford health care for your child, think again. Federal and state assistance programs through the Insure Kids Now Initiative now offer fairly comprehensive insurance for children of low-income families for as little as five dollars a month.

When you change work or can't work

After parting company with a company, workers used to find that their insurance was promptly cancelled, leaving them to fend for themselves. When they would begin a new job, their preexisting illnesses often weren't covered at all or at least for a portion of time. Because of this, many people stayed in unfulfilling, miserable jobs just to keep the insurance.

A couple of relatively new laws helped to change that scenario for Americans. First, the Consolidated Omnibus Budget Reconciliation Act (COBRA) of 1985 mandates that employers who offer a group health insurance plan to employees must continue to offer the option of insurance at the former employee's expense for up to eighteen months after employment ends. The cost assessed to the former employee can be 100 percent of the cost to the individual's portion of the group insurance plus 2 percent of that amount as an administrative fee. The former employee has sixty days after their final workday to make a decision regarding COBRA, leaving time to shop for individual insurance.

A newer law, the Health Insurance Portability and Accountability Act (HIPAA) of 1996, was primarily created to allow workers to change or lose their jobs without the threats to their continuing health insurance coverage. That is because the law limits the insurance companies' ability to exclude individuals with preexisting medical conditions from coverage or to refuse to issue or renew coverage if that individual was covered under a group plan for one full year immediately prior. Another bonus of the act is that it kicks in after COBRA coverage runs out, allowing the employee to renew the contract as an individual without the penalties normally associated with preexisting illnesses.

Practically speaking, the law allows an individual with IBD to continue coverage of their illness if they switch jobs, provided that they can prove that they were covered under a group plan for a certain amount of time after they were diagnosed with the illness. Previously, a new health plan enrollee would have their condition excluded from coverage for at least one year. With the law, the coverage would continue seamlessly.

Sometimes, IBD can be severe enough for the individual to have to cease working entirely or at least for a period of time. The U.S. government provides a safety net of sorts through Social Security.

One type of assistance, known as Social Security Disability Insurance (SSDI), is for individuals who have worked in the recent past and have paid Social Security taxes; another type, Social Security Insurance (SSI) is for individuals who haven't worked in a long time, if at all, and aren't eligible under SSDI guidelines. The benefits are only for those who have a diagnosed illness, physical or mental in nature, that makes working impossible for the current year and will remain so for the coming year. Both CD and UC are listed as diseases that can cause disability and medical requirements for determining the qualification of such have been identified by the government.

To qualify for these benefits, an individual has to embark on a lengthy application process. First, the individual has to apply for the benefit. In almost 70 percent of the cases, that application is turned down on the first try; however, an appeal can be heard by an administrative law judge within sixty days of the refusal. If that appeal is lost, another appeal can be filed in the same time frame to be heard by the Social Security Appeals Council in Arlington, Virginia. If that effort is lost, a further appeal can be filed in the same time frame with the U.S. District Court. If the appeal is won along the way or the application is granted on the first pass, the coverage is retroactive from the date of the disability.

Some say the most effective way to handle the appeals process is to retain an attorney who specializes in Social Security disability law. Generally, this is done on a contingency basis, with the lawyer recouping his or her fee if the case is won; then the amount of the fee is limited by law to 25 percent of the total. Fees relating to the obtaining of medical records and the like are deducted from the settlement separately.

Fighting back

There may be times when coverage of a procedure is denied by health insurance companies, or when other insurance benefits are not forthcoming when the intended recipient is entitled to them. There is almost always a way to redress these grievances through the insurance companies themselves or through a courtroom venue.

The first thing that should be done is to read the insurance policy to find out the proper procedure for filing a grievance or challenging a decision regarding care. In many cases, there is a specific individual or office within the insurance company that must be contacted. A form may have to be filled out and filed or perhaps the inquiry must be made in writing or through a personal telephone call. In any case, it may be helpful to keep copies of all correspondence coming in or going out. If phone calls are made, it may be useful to record the name of the individual spoken to as well as the time, date, and content of the call. If a call is made, request that a written reply be made to you as well to provide documentation of the call's content. Gathering all relevant medical records may also be of help. At the company with which you are employed, contact the benefits representative to let them in on the continuing discussions.

If there is a continued refusal of benefits, many insurance companies offer the option of appeal. This appeal is usually done in-house and may require the presence of the individual making the appeal. In most cases, the decision regarding the appeal will be issued in writing, specifying in detail the reasons to support the decision.

If the issue remains unresolved, there are a number of recourses short of filing a lawsuit. Although each state is different, the state's attorney general will likely investigate denial of coverage claims and can force the insurer to comply. A state's medical society can work with the doctor to explain the reasoning behind the procedures and the necessity and appropriateness of coverage to the insurance company. Legal aid societies often have insurance departments that can help to negotiate the coverage free of charge.

When all else has failed, many individuals have sued the insurance companies and won, forcing the coverage. It is important to find a lawyer who specializes in health care law to do so and to be prepared for a lengthy fight.

Some insurance do's and don'ts

○ Do learn as much as possible about the disease, what is required in care, and what treatment options are commonly used. You may have to explain this someday to your benefits representative or may have to know it in case of a dispute over charges.

○ Do read the insurance policy in its entirety. Loopholes can limit coverage or do away with it entirely in certain situations. Know what the policy covers.

○ Do keep copies of all policies in a safe location.

○ Do ask questions. Make sure that you fully understand all of the coverage.

○ Don't be late in your payments or allow the policy to lapse.

○ Don't buy insurance from a newspaper advertisement or from a sign on the side of the road. Most of those plans do not offer adequate coverage for IBD-related concerns.

IN A SENTENCE:

> *Insurance of all kinds is available and important, and every effort should be made to understand coverage.*

Children and IBD

HAVING A chronic illness is a difficult load to bear for most adults but for children with chronic illness, that load can be particularly exquisite. That is because a child is still beginning to form a sense of him- or herself, and having to deal with a chronic illness during these precarious phases of development can be trying. Add to this the body-morphing and mentally disquieting effects of certain IBD medications, the isolation of hospitalizations, and the pain and fatigue associated with the conditions, and it is somewhat amazing that many of the children with IBD have positive attitudes at all.

When that is the case, give some credit to the parents and guardians behind those children. These individuals have helped these children navigate not only the traditional trials and tribulations of childhood and adolescence, but they have also helped them to successfully negotiate the twists and turns that chronic illness throws into life. Ask these adults what the secret is and they will tell you that it has to do with patience, determination, and ardent advocacy on their child's behalf.

Alterations in home life

Perhaps the first hurdle parents face in dealing with the needs of a child with a chronic illness comes in educating the child, other family members, and friends about the illness. To be well-armed with information means gathering pamphlets and books about IBD and visiting websites. A bonus in this search for knowledge to share is that you, too, will become educated; the more equipped with knowledge you are, the less scary the diseases will be, the more in control you will feel about some of the treatments and the better you will be at noticing signs of intestinal or extraintestinal manifestations of the disease when the child cannot.

Peggy, a CD patient with nineteen-year-old twin daughters both diagnosed with UC, says educating yourself is perhaps the best thing a parent of an IBD patient can do for their child.

"Educate yourself as much as possible. There is a lot of information available, especially since we have the Internet in our homes and libraries. Research about the disease itself and the medications your child is on. Search, search, and search some more for all the information you can find," she said. However, she cautions that not all information is reliable or accurate, especially on the Internet, where some sites simply seek to sell products. "Medical Web sites are great sources. I can't stress enough how being educated about the disease itself has helped us. I have been able to download medical studies, print them out, and present them to our doctor. And he has been more willing to try things when he sees that it is from a reliable medical source or study."

Consult with the physician about the best way to tell the child if the child has not already been told. Doctors are used to breaking such news to their patients and may have some tips or helpful materials to share with you. Children should be told about the disease, but spare the gory details or in-depth knowledge for when they are best able to handle them. Let them know that you are there to help them and will be with them throughout the treatment of the disease.

When explaining the disease to others within the immediate family, speak in terms that they can understand. For a younger sibling, you may want to tell them that their brother or sister has stomachaches and diarrhea (something many children can relate with) but that they can't catch this illness. Be sure to keep medication out of their reach. Other family members should be told about the illness and should be warned that the child may need to use the bathroom more urgently, allowing them to have permanent "dibs" on the bathroom.

As a parent, you may also want to take advantage of the support options detailed in Day 4. This is especially true if you feel fear or uncertainty about your child's illness. For many children, sensing fear in their parents translates to greater fear in themselves. Dealing with your feelings in a positive venue such as a Web board for parents of children with IBD, out of sight of your child, will help both of you.

Mike found this to be a source of comfort. The father of a young adult with UC, he regularly posts on dragonpack.com, a site for the parents of other IBD patients. "Become an expert on your child's disease and continue to communicate with those who've been through the war," he said. "They are a tremendous source of encouragement, knowledge, and comfort."

Food issues of the child may well become issues for the family, as the preparation of meals may involve taking into consideration foods or substances that can promote diarrhea. Bonnie, the mother of David, a CD patient, said that she began to pack his lunch more for school to avoid higher fat items on the school's menu and made other alterations to accommodate the illness.

"We do not eat at fast food places like we used to, which is better for all of us. Now David will choose Subway instead of McDonald's," she said. "We make healthy choices. Instead of French fries, David will go with a baked potato. We do not eat red meat as much as we did in the past."

Perhaps the biggest change in the home life will be establishing a regular schedule for medication to be administered and then administering. Many of the medications available for the treatment of IBD in adults are used in children, despite the fact that most of the drugs have not been thoroughly studied for use in the pediatric population. Also, many of the drugs available are not made in kid-friendly, good-tasting suspension formulas, like the bubblegum-flavored ubiquitous amoxicillin for many childhood illnesses; that said, major drugstore chains like CVS and Rite Aid will provide palatable flavorings to children's liquid medicine for a small surcharge. For those having to use enema preparations or having to have nasogastric feedings, the struggle can become more physical in nature as foreign objects are inserted into uncomfortable areas.

For medication, there are a few tricks for getting kids to take it. First, it is important to establish that the medication is a necessity, not simply a way to torture the child. If the child understands that the medication will help to control the bad symptoms, he or she may be more likely to take the medication without a struggle.

Karen, the mother of four-year-old CD patient Kate, equated the taking of the medication to the use of the car seat.

"It is just going to happen. We don't beg and cajole, or try to sweet talk her into it. We have explained from the beginning that the medicine is good for her, and she has to have it to make her tummy feel better," Karen said. "Kate knows that it is a completely nonnegotiable issue, and has always been very good about it."

If the medication is in a pill form that can be ground up (for example, prednisone is one of these drugs, Pentasa capsules can be opened, but Asacol tablets shouldn't be broken), it can be mixed with something sweet like a spoonful of honey, yogurt, or applesauce. Yucky suspension liquids can be squirted directly down the throat or placed in the cheek; coating the tongue with a tiny bit of peanut butter, honey, or chocolate sauce first or immediately afterward can help to ward off or diminish the bad taste. When a child is old enough to swallow the pills, allow them to pick a liquid to down them with. Don't wince if that liquid is Pepsi and it is 7 A.M.; allowing them some control or choice in the matter will make taking medication less awful.

For Karen, teaching her daughter to swallow pills was an effort in and of itself. Beginning at the age of two, Karen began having her daughter try swallowing Jell-O Jigglers without chewing them. When Kate accomplished this task, Karen would make a slit in the Jiggler and place the pill in it. Soon after, Kate learned to swallow the small pills without the Jell-O.

For enemas or nasogastric tubes, it is important to get some instruction from the child's health care provider first. These individuals—either doctors or nurses—have likely instructed many other families on this issue and may have some helpful hints to share. To make this time easier for the child, it may be helpful for them to have some self-selected source of comfort or distraction such as a favorite stuffed animal, movie, or a video game.

As the child becomes more proficient in handling the matter themselves, you can hand over this responsibility, checking only that they didn't dump the enema or feeding material in the toilet.

Many of the medications that must be taken for the treatment of the disease must be done at a few intervals during the day. Mealtimes and bedtimes are easy to remember. As the child gets older and begins to take the medication with less of your help, buy them something to remind them of the medication schedule such as a watch with an alarm or a small, portable pill box with an alarm. For more information on such products, see Week 3. Peer pressure increases as the child ages, leaving many adolescents to hide or "forget" to take medication in an effort to be more like their peers, most of whom will not have to take regular medication. The best weapon against this is education, which can be accomplished by explaining how each medication works and why it is important to take that medication regularly.

Selecting the health care team

The major difference between selecting the health care team for an adult and doing the same for the child is that the decisions you make will affect two or more people, the parent(s) and the child. Because this is the case, be sure to ask the same questions as in Day 5 but also be sure to find a doctor who you can respect and who will respect your role as a parent.

That doesn't mean you will crowd the doctors, making it impossible for them to do their jobs. Instead, you and the doctors will work as a team, you as the expert on your child and the doctors as the experts in the disease and its treatment.

"Don't be intimidated by the doctor," said Karen. "Their job is to make your child feel better and they should do this by working with you, as the expert on your own child. Maybe parents aren't the experts on the disease but they certainly are the experts on how their child feels. I think that the level of concern a mom feels in her gut is something to be taken very seriously because something can just look or feel wrong to the parents before it is obvious to the doctor.

"That has happened with us many times, and we take our own concerns seriously and expect our doctor to as well," she continued.

Out and about with IBD

Leaving the home with someone who is dependent upon a bathroom may seem tricky but can be done with ease, provided some planning is done in advance. Before leaving on local trips, be sure to have your child make a bathroom stop to try to go. Also, it might be wise during flare-ups to carry an extra change of clothes in the trunk or in a backpack just in case.

When you are out in public and your opposite sex, younger child needs to use the restroom, it is okay to take them into your sex-appropriate bathroom to take care of their needs. If a problem should arise, quietly discuss the issue with a manager. Ignore any busybody who should approach you on the issue, as it is clearly none of their business. When traveling with a child, the same tips and suggestions for adult travel covered in Month 9 apply.

Perhaps the greatest care you should take with your child is in preparing them for surviving the school situation. This is because teachers and administrators should know about your child's chronic condition in order to make allowances such as extra bathroom breaks, excuses from gym activities when the child is not feeling well, and a system for gathering homework assignments when the child is too ill to attend school.

For all concerned, it is best to make these arrangements as soon as possible. This is because all kinds of assumptions can be made regarding the behavior of the child. For example, a child who uses the bathroom in excess of others might be seen as goofing off while a child who is absent a lot may be seen as being truant, especially if the child looks well. Also, some schools lock the bathrooms while class is in session to prevent dawdlers while others remove the stall doors of the individual bathrooms to take any hideouts away from wayward smokers. Further, the side effects of such drugs as prednisone can make the child less than cooperative in a classroom setting.

It is best to make an appointment with the administrators and the child's teachers to explain the situation to them. Prior to the meeting, you may want to contact the local CCFA chapter for brochures and other educational materials to hand out. At the appointment, explain the disease and how it works, being sure to emphasize that while the child may look well, he or she may also be experiencing symptoms. Then tell the administrators and teachers how this might affect your child during school hours when the child is in their care. Try to come up with solutions, such as a hand signal that lets the teacher know the child needs to exit immediately to use the bathroom or allow access to the teachers' bathrooms where stall doors aren't an issue.

Lindsey, who has CD, teaches at a school in Michigan. She routinely tells her fifth grade students that she has the disease as a way to explain any unforeseen absences in the school year. She believes that the meeting with parents and administrators should also involve the child.

"As a teacher, we are better suited to meet the needs of children when we know what is occurring in their personal lives, because kids can't learn and cannot focus on something when their mind is focused on how they can leave the room for the eighth time to go to the bathroom without getting in trouble," she said. "It is not an easy conversation but it is one that the child, not just the parent, needs to have with the teacher. Teachers are very accommodating when they know what they are dealing with. After I shared my story with my students, I found out that one of them has it as well, and we have worked out a system for leaving the room. [We have] been a support for one another when either isn't feeling well."

Another issue for children with IBD in the school setting arises when the child is on immunosuppressant medication. Schools are notorious germ havens because many children haven't mastered good hygiene or are so close to one another that it is impossible not to share colds and other airborne illnesses. For this reason, it is important that the child is protected from communicable illnesses by receiving vaccines for illnesses such as chicken pox or by receiving the annual flu shot. Additionally, good hygiene including frequent hand washing can prevent some of these illnesses from starting. Because schools at times are not stocked with adequate supplies of soap and paper towels, it might be a good idea to supply the teacher or the child with liquid hand sanitizer.

Helping Children Survive the hospital

Hospitals are scary, lonely places for adults. This can be doubly so for a child who is in pain and may have never slept away from home for more than a night. Even though hospitals have come a long way in creating colorful playrooms and crazy clothing for the health care providers, a hospital is still not home, a message that comes across over and over with every needle stick that is felt and every IV pole that is seen.

To make a hospital room a more comforting place to be, consider bringing in some of the comforts of home that the child normally enjoys. A favorite blanket, their own pillow, and their favorite toy can help to create a more comfortable, familiar area.

When David was hospitalized three times before a diagnosis was made, Bonnie made sure to bring in magazines and books for him to read, as well as his own pillow and photographs of family members and favorite pets.

"My husband and I were with him as much as possible when he was admitted. It is a scary thing to be away from family, sick, lonely, not knowing what is wrong. We just try to ease the tension as much as possible," she said. "Of course, I am totally exhausted by the time he is discharged and need a vacation, but we do what we have to do for our children!"

If a child is small and afraid of being alone, hospitals almost always allow a parent or guardian to stay with them through the night (usually on a chair that converts to a bed) and accompany them to all of the procedures during the day. Doing this helps to relieve the stress on both the child and the parent. In most cases, the hospital allows the parents to use a shower and to order meals through the hospital kitchen for a nominal fee. It helps to rotate the parents doing hospital duty or have other loving relatives step in to give Mom and Dad a break.

Financing the illness

The price of medications, surgeries, and other illness-associated costs strap many families. And yet, without the treatment, the child would likely suffer a worse fate. However, there are some avenues through which costs can be cut or other assistance can be found.

As stated in Month 9, every state boasts a cheap insurance program specifically designed for children. Also, many states offer other programs for aid in buying medication. A hospital financial aid representative should have information on those programs. For medication, doctors often have ample supplies of free trial packs of some of the brand name medications such as Asacol or Pentasa. Pharmaceutical companies also have specific programs for reduced cost medication for low-income families. Your child's doctor should be able to help you with information in that regard.

Doctors can and do waive fees at times for a variety of reasons. When this is not possible, a discussion with the office manager regarding a payment schedule can help to distribute large costs over a longer period of time, making the bills more manageable. Hospitals often do the same thing.

Peggy has a unique solution for dealing with the insurance companies. "Make friends at your insurance company with someone who you can call for assistance. You can't always do that with a big company, but be friendly and cheerful and you will be amazed at how far it can get you," she said. "Call them by name, treat them like they are friends, because they are. They are the ones that can help you when you really need it. Once, I sent a dozen bagels to the representative at our insurance company in Nevada (we are in California). It cost me forty-five dollars to send it via next day air but she really appreciated it. She remembers me when I call and always takes good care of me, telling me 'anything you need.' I have saved at least a thousand dollars since I spent that forty-five dollars. It was well worth it."

CCFA Camp Oasis

Every kid needs to be a kid, especially those who face chronic illnesses. Going on that belief, the Crohn's & Colitis Foundation of America sponsors a summer camp program that now boasts nine different sites. In these camps, children from seven to eighteen years in age swap stories over the nightly campfire, learn archery, ride horses, play water sports, perform in talent shows, do arts and crafts projects, and, perhaps most importantly, meet other kids who also struggle with IBD.

The camps, usually four to six days in length, are generally free, although parents with children in some camps have to pay any long distance travel to the camp. There is also a nominal application fee and scholarship money to cover that cost when necessary.

The camps are staffed around the clock with doctors, nurses, and other health care providers familiar with the diseases, as well as specially trained and screened counselors. For more information about the camps, visit the CCFA Web site at www.ccfa.org.

IN A SENTENCE:

Raising a child with IBD presents its own challenges in terms of school, hospitalizations, costs, and daily activities.

learning

Treatments for Children with IBD

MUCH OF what has already been covered in this book regarding treatment for IBD applies to children. However, children have special concerns regarding the diseases and their treatments, as they are still growing.

Symptoms and diagnosis

The symptoms of UC and CD are the same in children as they are in adults, as is the diagnostic process. A difference may exist in children when they don't give a voice to the symptoms, thinking some of the manifestations of the illness are normal bowel patterns or being embarrassed to discuss changes in bowel habits. Also, smaller children may not be able to tell a parent or guardian where it hurts or what is different. For these children, fever, weight loss, or lack of growth may be the biggest indicators of disease activity.

A pediatrician or a parent may notice the symptoms, leading to the same series of diagnostic tests and procedures that an adult with similar symptoms would undergo. One difference in the diagnostic process is that the pediatrician or pediatric gastroenterologist will have to rule out other, child-specific illnesses such as in certain babies who have immunological conditions, the symptoms of which mimic colitis. Other organ system problems also have to be taken into account and may lead to tests on the heart, kidneys, or other organs. For example, the first symptom may be swollen ankles, leading to blood tests for kidney failure.

The actual tests are calibrated for the size of the patient, and even the littlest of patients can undergo the same tests as full-sized adults. One example of this is the colonoscopy. In recent years, smaller, thinner pediatric endoscopy equipment has become standard in hospital endoscopy suites, and anesthetic techniques have been developed to minimize any pain to infants, children, and adolescents with minimum side effects.

Medication and surgery

Once the child is diagnosed with IBD, the treatments are the same as their adult counterparts. But while children are often prescribed these medications, there usually exist no large-scale studies on the effects and the most effective dosages for children.

This lack of testing is despite the large numbers of individuals under the age of eighteen who have the disease; according to one report, it is estimated that one-tenth of IBD patients or 100,000 to 140,000 children in America have been diagnosed with and are receiving treatment for IBD. It is also despite a push of the drug companies by the U.S. Food and Drug Administration to do more such studies for the safety and efficacy of medications administered to the pediatric population. One understandable snag in this effort is that many parents aren't willing to put their children up as medication study subjects.

That said, the greatest concern with medical therapy in children is the use of medications that can affect the growth of the child. Children with IBD may already be of a shorter stature than their healthier counterparts due to decreased absorption and nutrition issues. To complicate matters, steroids are often prescribed to rein in the inflammatory process of the disease. One undesirable side effect of steroids such as prednisone and prednisolone in children is that it hampers normal growth, a nonissue in adult-onset CD and UC because full height has often already been achieved. Because of this, steroids are often used for the shortest terms possible, with greater use of immunosuppressant medication to avoid these effects.

For surgical intervention, stress is placed on minimalist approaches, especially in the case of CD patients. A child diagnosed with CD will have the disease for a lifetime and will often require repeat surgeries. Thus, the less intestine removed, the better.

Nutrition and growth issues

While controlling the illnesses with medication and surgery are paramount in children, an equally important aspect of IBD care in children will involve the maintenance of normal growth and development. Normal growth in healthy children requires the intake of more calories, especially for children who are active in sports or other physically demanding activities such as dance, and disease activity itself requires greater energy on the part of the body. If children are shying away from food in the first place due to the way it makes them feel, they will likely experience a bigger deficit. Usually, this is of greater importance in children with CD in the small intestine, as this can impair proper absorption of nutrients. Children with UC can also have growth and nutrition issues due to lessened intake attributed to nausea or pain.

When these situations occur, the doctor may ask that the child consult with a nutritionist or registered dietitian to find an acceptable way to increase caloric consumption. Through a proper diet, perhaps with extra snacks, additions of nutritionally sound drinks such as protein shakes or Boost, or more meals in a day, the child may be able to catch up to normal growth levels.

When this is not effective, a doctor may prescribe nasogastric night feedings of an elemental formula. Usually, this formula can be ingested in the normal way but the taste is often unpalatable for children, making the tube feeding the only alternative. To do this, the child or the parent learns to insert the tube up through the nose and down the throat into the stomach each night. A bag of prepared formula is attached to a pump that slowly administers the formula as the child sleeps, adding thousands of nutritionally complete calories to help feed the body for growth. Often, this is done for a few months until the child is able to grow to expected levels.

IN A SENTENCE:

> *Medical and surgical treatment of IBD in children is nearly the same as it is for adults.*

Understanding Research

NEWS STORIES about breakthroughs in medical research are written all of the time, usually with great fanfare. When the artificial heart was implanted in one and then another and another patient, the television news media dedicated whole programs to the creation of the device. Less spectacular advances also regularly grab headlines, news that brings joy to the hearts of investors and patients internationally. If such an article detailing the advances of research in IBD appeared in the months since your diagnosis, you probably paid a great deal of attention to it.

Although the viewers and readers of the news may be familiar with the medical stories, few outside of the medical profession know the difference between what a Phase III drug has gone through as opposed to one in a Phase I trial. Because of this, doctors are usually inundated with copies of stories touting the miracle that twelve patients in a Phase I trial experienced in terms of reversal of IBD symptoms, given to them by patients who want to know why they don't have access to that same medication.

By understanding the different steps in medical research and most especially drug research, patients can not only have a better grasp on the relevance of a media story about an advance, but they can also keep tabs on promising medicines and technology. Knowing about which drugs are in development can also allow some patients to participate in the research process by becoming a study subject.

The beginning of clinical drug research

As with all great things, a drug begins with an idea. A research scientist or doctor who is involved in research may put forth a hypothesis about what causes a disease or acts as a participant in a crucial process that occurs in the disease. Sometimes, that idea is based on original research, other times it is inspired by the findings of another researcher or team of researchers at a hospital or university. With IBD, an obvious and fertile area of interest is the inflammatory process. In that area, a scientist might become interested in studying some of the cellular interactions in the early stages of inflammation, for example. This focus will center on trying to find a way to halt the process by inhibiting different cellular reactions. That researcher would then develop a natural or synthetic material that would act to inhibit the cells from participating in inflammation. Additionally, a delivery method (i.e., intramuscular injection or pill) would be created to best bring the drug to the essential site.

But just because the medication appears ready for human ingestion, it is not. It first has to be proven to be safe and effective for the purpose through administration to an animal. Labs generally use different kinds of animals since the medications can have different effects on the different species. Rats, cats, mice, dogs, and chimpanzees are often the subjects of such tests and are carefully and humanely cared for during the time of research. The animals are then given the treatment, after which their blood levels and other metabolic reactions are closely monitored. Many times, this research continues after human trials have commenced to monitor the long-term effects of the drugs.

While many of the drugs tested never make it past the animal trials, a fraction of them do, opening the door to formal testing on humans. At this stage, a manufacturer has to fill out an investigational new drug (IND) application that is submitted to the U.S. Food and Drug Administration's

(FDA) Center for Drug Evaluation and Research. This application includes information on the results of animal testing, the chemical composition of the drug, toxicology information, company and production information, and design of the proposed study. Of particular interest to the FDA is the study's commitment to follow government safety requirements for the research participants. The FDA then reviews the applications and renders a decision regarding approval or disapproval within thirty days of the receipt of the application.

Phases of a study

Assuming the application passes review, the human testing can begin in clinical trials. In the first phase of the trials, the researchers gather anywhere from a half dozen to several dozen patients and healthy individuals who agree to use the drug for a certain period of time, usually less than a year. The individuals report to the researchers at regular intervals to have their blood levels measured and to talk about their reactions to the drugs. In these Phase I trials, the participants are often aware of what the drug is and what its intended use is.

All of the information from this first trial is gathered. Recorded in the information is how the body metabolizes and/or absorbs the drug, how the body gets rid of the drug, what side effects occur at what dose, what the most tolerable dose of the drug is before intolerable side effects occur, as well as the number and kinds of side effects experienced by the research participants. If a large amount of the information is deemed too negative to move forward, the clinical testing stops there.

However, if the greater amount is positive, the second phase of the study begins; about 70 percent of the initial drugs that participate in Phase I move on to Phase II. In this phase, only patients who would stand to benefit from the medication, i.e., IBD patients for IBD drugs, are recruited as test subjects. The patient body numbers usually in the hundreds, with more than one site recruited to perform the research. Phase II trials last anywhere from several months to two years. Information regarding short-term effectiveness and safety is gathered from this phase and will determine whether the clinical trials will advance to Phase III trials.

At this stage in the game, about one third of the original IND drug applications will still be in the running for approval. Here, several hundred to several thousand individuals who will potentially benefit from such a medication participate in the same research protocols at several centers. This phase is the true proving ground as it is at this stage where the drug is compared with other drugs and different dosages are tested for effectiveness and safety. This stage is typically the longest, lasting one to four years.

About 25 to 30 percent of the original IND applicants make it past the third stage with positive results. The drug companies then gather all of the research data and present it to the FDA in the form of a new drug application (NDA). The companies then wait anywhere from six to ten months for a FDA panel to analyze the data. The FDA can then choose whether or not it will approve the drug for marketing; at times, the FDA will make marketing suggestions that must be adhered to before the drug makes it to the pharmacy shelves. According to the FDA, about 20 percent of the original IND applicants go on to final marketing.

Different elements of studies

Generally speaking, the farther the study gets, the greater degree of complexity is involved. While every participant of the first stage of the trial will likely know what they are getting (called "open label") and why they are getting it, those toward the tail end of the study may know what the drug is, but they may not be sure they are getting the drug at all.

After Phase I is completed and larger groups of test subjects are recruited, the participants generally are assigned to a varying amounts of control groups. In some studies, the patients receive one dose of the medication while the others receive a placebo, an inert substance. In other studies, three groups exist: one that gets a standard dose, one that receives another level of the drug, and the third that receives the placebo. This helps the researchers to determine whether patients are receiving a benefit of the drug over the placebo group's results, and at which level of dosage the drug is the most efficacious.

Sometimes, the groups switch treatment halfway through the testing. This allows the researchers to see if the groups respond equally to the different controls. For example, in one recent study, participants were separated into two groups. The first group received the treatment for one year and the second group received the placebo for the same amount of time. In the second year of the study, those receiving the treatment got the placebo while those who had the placebo began receiving the treatment. It was found that during the time the patients received the treatment, they fared better, experiencing fewer symptoms than when they were on the placebo.

To say that a control group is double-blind does not mean that they are without sight in both eyes. Instead, it means that neither the researchers nor the patients know to which group they have been assigned. Usually, an administrator assigns a code to each patient so only the administrator knows who has been assigned to which group. The reasons for a double-blind trial are many, but the most important is that the participants and the researchers will not be able to color their judgment of the positive or negative effect of the drug, because no one but the administrator is sure who is receiving what.

When a study is said to be randomized, that means that the patients have been randomly assigned, regardless of their ages, sex, and severity of their illness. This measure prevents unscrupulous researchers from unfairly loading the results of the study by using relatively well patients or those who would benefit most from the drug, thus rendering glowing results. If a trial is said to be "multicentered," then that means that more than one research facility (i.e., hospitals, universities, doctors' offices, independent labs) are used to duplicate the protocols. This is done to facilitate the larger numbers of participants and to show that the results can be reproduced.

Paying for the research

Initially, drug companies must put forth a great deal of money to fund the research of the medications. According to governmental data from 1993, drug companies shell out $359 million to develop one drug, from conception to pharmacy shelves. This money pays for the lab time of the researchers, the physicians and researchers to administer the phases of the tests, the production of the test medicine, and the information gathering. Certainly, many hands are involved in the testing of a medication, and all of those hands are paid salaries as well.

But the drug companies, while the initial sponsors of the trials, are not funding the trials out of the goodness of their hearts. Those costs are passed on to you, the consumer. That is why, for example, an allergy drug can cost you $120 for one month's prescription. It is not that the compound in the capsule is so rare; rather, all of the costs of the research are recouped through the sales of the medication.

While it would seem that it would be more advantageous to the consumer to purchase a generic form of the drug, often that is not possible since laws protect the drug patents for a certain amount of time, assuring the companies that a cheaper version of the drug can't be produced as they recoup their research dollars and squeeze out a profit.

Some drug companies also take advantage of the Orphan Drug Act of 1983. This act was designed to promote the creation of drugs for rare diseases for which there previously had been little incentive to create these medications. For example, a medication for proctitis may only see 50,000 to 100,000 patients using the drug during their lifetime as opposed to a drug for rheumatoid arthritis, which has a potential consumer base of several million sufferers.

To qualify for orphan drug status, a drug must be designed for the needs of a disease that strikes fewer than 200,000 Americans. UC and CD are considered diseases that qualify for orphan drug status even though 500,000 Americans are affected by each disease, because certain manifestations of the diseases affect less than the 200,000 threshold. The benefits of attaining the orphan drug status is that the companies can apply for grant money to reduce some of the research costs, tax breaks are awarded to those companies participating in orphan drug research, application fees are waived, and research design assistance is offered free of charge. The result of the passing of the act has been a rapid increase in the number of drugs developed to treat rare diseases in the United States.

Other kinds of research

One needs to look no further than medical journals to know that medication isn't the only area of research that is done. Other major breakthroughs in the understanding of disease activity are found on a daily basis in labs across the country and around the world. This is the type of research that garners Nobel Prizes and other major accolades.

In UC and CD research, for example, researchers continue to look into the genetic component of the diseases, as well as cellular interactions and other areas. The research may involve registries of hundreds of individuals, or a few biopsy specimens taken during colonoscopies. The researchers make hypotheses, set up the design of the study, gather their data and attempt to publish their findings in notable journals. This information is presented time and again at medical conferences and other professional gatherings.

Commonly, this research is funded through grants from the government or from private entities such as the CCFA and is supported by universities and hospitals. The government, through the National Institutes of Health, funds thousands of these studies each year. A much smaller number of grants are issued by CCFA for similar research projects.

IN A SENTENCE:

> Research is a lengthy and complicated process that should be understood by all people who have IBD.

living

Participating in Research

MAYBE YOUR disease is in a severe stage and nothing is working, or perhaps the available options aren't right because you are allergic to them. Or maybe you want to participate more fully in finding a cure. Whatever the reason, you may be a candidate to participate in a clinical research trial.

Finding information on trials

Your first stop for information on clinical trials should be your doctor. This individual will likely be aware of the research going on in a hospital or university within close proximity to where you live. He or she may be conducting research as well, or be a colleague of someone who is doing so. They are also usually the recipient of information regarding trials that are looking for volunteers or physician participants.

If you are looking to get into a trial because you need another avenue of treatment, this discussion with your doctor should include information on what your current FDA-approved treatment options are. Be wary of dismissing any approved and proven treatments in favor of trial medication with unknown side effects; clinical trial options do not have fully documented side effects, safety, or efficacy. An example of this would be to forgo prednisone for an experimental medication, the side effects of which are not completely known at this point. Also, realize that you may not get the drug and instead be treated with a placebo.

Discuss with your doctor whether your current condition and needs fit the protocol of the study. As an example, one drug study in which I contemplated participating had a protocol that insisted participants not become pregnant during the year of the study and mandated that those participating promise to use two forms of birth control and submit to regular pregnancy testing. Obviously, I was sick enough that pregnancy was not a good option at the time, but for others who were contemplating pregnancy, this drug study would not have been for them.

Another part of the discussion should include how far you are willing to go to be a participant in the study. This means distance and inconvenience. You may be willing to drive to and from a research facility located 200 miles from your home once, but are you willing to do so eight to twelve times during the course of the study? Are you willing to inject yourself with the medication? Are you willing to undergo either planned hospitalization for procedures or unplanned hospitalization for severe side effects? All of these questions should be answered ahead of time.

If your doctor is not aware of drug studies in the immediate or not too distant area, seek the information on your own. The best place for this information is on the Internet. Most research facilities—hospitals and universities—host websites that include information regarding ongoing research projects and places where you can request more information. If the site has not been updated in a while, a phone call to the research coordinators or administrators at these facilities can be a source for more current information.

There are also a few reliable websites that serve the public and the research facilities by offering a place to read and to post information about the clinical trials.

O The information at www.centerwatch.com includes tens of thousands of industry- and government-sponsored clinical trials as well as information about new drugs, the laboratories conducting the studies, and general information about research. For information about IBD drugs, visit the gastroenterology section under the trial listings section.

○ The National Institutes of Health sponsors the listings at www.clinicaltrials.gov. To find information on UC or CD trials, browse the trials by condition, which are listed alphabetically.

○ Sponsored by a number of drug companies, a private company hosts www.Acurian.com. This site contains thousands of listings of current clinical trials, separated by condition and by location with links to websites for more information about trials.

○ On its Web site, the CCFA has a list of clinical trials for IBD with links or contact information. Visit the main site at www.ccfa.org.

If the protocol for the trial is not listed on the site, contact the clinical trial administrator and request a copy of the protocol.

Participating in clinical trials

Once you have reviewed the protocol and feel you can comply with it, you should then contact the research administrator to volunteer. Likely, a discussion will follow regarding the protocol for the trial and whether you fit the criteria to participate as a volunteer.

Paperwork will then be sent to your home or through e-mail. Other than a map for the facility, a welcome letter, and instructions, the packet you receive should include a special agreement called an informed consent. This document, usually several pages in length, contains information about the drug and its possible benefits as well as the purpose of the research. You will find out here how long your participation will be, how many doctor or research visits are required, and whether any hospitalization is required as well as other treatments that are available currently outside of the clinical trial option. The informed consent will give you some idea of the risks you face in taking the unproven medication or treatment, what will happen if the effects are bad enough to require hospitalization and who or what entity will be responsible for covering those costs. There will be contact information for the administrator and for others who can help you during the trial at a time of crisis such as a doctor familiar with the trial. Finally, it should tell you that your records will be kept confidential and that your participation is voluntary at all times. If you don't understand the information in the

Creating Restroom Access Legislation

Not long after the publication of the first edition of this book, I began to have severe symptoms again. Fevers, bleeding, weight loss, and abdominal pain became a constant presence in my life, forcing me to slow down in a way in which I was not comfortable. I had been through all of the treatment options available, including Remicade, an infusion of which led to a serum-sickness reaction and a life threatening infection. So I did what many people would do in my position: I entered a medical trial for a new medication.

After consulting with my gastroenterologist, I searched my immediate area for open trials and found one that looked promising: an infusion drug for people with moderate to severe CD that was being tested in a hospital in Detroit about fifteen miles from my home. I met with the study coordinator, a nurse who interviewed me at length, and then with the site's principal coordinator, a gastroenterologist who provided care for me during the trial. They explained that I would be randomly assigned to one of two groups, receiving either the placebo or the medication. They also said I would receive infusions a few hours at a time, three days a week for four weeks for a total of twelve infusions. Within a week of our initial meeting, I had gone through a thorough exam, signed the informed consent, and was cleared for the infusions.

During the first week, I suffered a bad reaction to the infusion, spiking a seemingly unshakable fever of 104 degrees for about eight hours and feeling intense flu-like symptoms. The doctor saw me the next day and said I could quit the trial if I wished. But I decided to go forward, taking the added measures of medicating with Benadryl and Tylenol before future infusions. Over a week, the reaction abated and I started to feel better. For the next several weeks, I transmitted personal information about my health to the investigators and continued to check in with the local contacts at the hospital. Though I felt better with the infusions, my participation ended when my annual colonoscopy showed a need for surgery due to a stricture caused by scar tissue.

Would I do it again? Yes. Though I suffered through a week of bad side effects, I received great care, felt some relief from my symptoms, and was able to help move science forward in a unique way, a factor that was important to me at the time.

Should you do it? Again, you are in charge of your medical decisions. Just as you should weigh all of your options before going on a new medication that is approved, you should also weigh all of your options before becoming a participant in a clinical trial for an unapproved medication.

informed consent, be sure to discuss this with the administrator before signing the informed consent and turning it in.

If this seems like a lot of information, get used to it, says Lynn. She is participating in a unique study for a treatment in her home state of Iowa. "I have to keep a weekly diary of all symptoms, i.e., general well-being, blood in stool, urgency, number of loose or liquid stools, abdominal pain/cramps, arthritis or joint pain, eye pain/redness, painful skin ulcers/red bumps/canker sores, anal fissure, fistula or abscess/drainage/opening/ulcers/collection of pus in the anal region, other fistula, fever over 100 degrees F during the previous seven days," she said. "I have to fill out questionnaires about my symptoms and quality of life, complete medical history, have a physical exam, and have a number of baseline tests done to determine my current physical condition."

The medication in the trial should come at no cost to you. If the treatment is successful and another phase or phases of the trials must still be completed before the medication is approved, there should be a way for you to continue to receive a "compassionate" prescription for the medication for a certain amount of time; some trials contain an open phase where the patients continue to receive the treatment as long as their condition continues to be monitored.

Before you begin the trial, you may be required to undergo a physical that is administered by a doctor who is participating in the trial. This initial consultation is a good time to talk about any concerns or questions you might have regarding the trial. Regular visits to plot your progress will be required, usually frequent at first with fewer toward the end of the trial. Be sure to keep these appointments as it allows the clinicians to record any side effects as well as any benefits.

Realize that you are not bound to continue the trial if you experience any amount of discomfort during the trial. This is a totally voluntary experience and you do not owe it to anyone to continue if you find it difficult to do so. Volunteers drop out of studies all the time for a variety of reasons. It should not be held against you to do so.

Also realize that the trial may end unexpectedly. Although this doesn't happen often, some trial administrators and researchers may conclude early on that the drug either has a significant benefit or deleterious effect for those using it. In the case of the benefit, the trial can be stopped so all participants can benefit from the drug. In the case where the drug shows that damage is being done to the participants who receive it, the trial can be stopped and the drug withdrawn.

As a participant in a trial, you can ask for a copy of the final findings. Usually, the trial administrator can send the information following publication of the material.

IN A SENTENCE:

> *Participating in a trial is manageable and rewarding when the process and requirements are understood.*

Moving On

IN THE past twelve months, your life has changed in at least one very significant way: you have a chronic illness. That illness is defined daily for you by the ingesting of a variety of medications, more frequent trips to the bathroom, or the occurrence of specific pain. This journey through tests and procedures, medicines, and perhaps surgeries likely has tried you physically, mentally, and emotionally. In so many ways, you are not the same person you were the minute before your diagnosis.

That isn't necessarily an entirely bad thing. It is through adversity that we grow and move forward. Perhaps you have a greater appreciation for being well or maybe you have met some wonderful people you may have never met without having this disease. Maybe you simply now know more about how your body works and how best to take care of it. And you might just have realized how precious and special your life really is through the love and concern others have shown you.

Throughout all of this, life goes on, and it will continue to do so. Now is the time to figure out where you are going to put this new baggage, the place for the CD or UC in your life. It likely won't always be front and center unless a medical emergency takes place. Instead, your life—all you want to experience, all you are, and all you want to become—should be a primary focus. It might have been hard to think about plans when the uncertainty of the disease was all about you. But there is no reason for you to be stopped in your tracks forever.

Define your life and your life goals

You have learned in the past year that life with CD and UC can be managed through medication and surgery coordinated by you and your health care team. Life's every day obstacles can be made manageable through the use of helpful tips and suggestions, as well as a good deal of planning. Knowing all of this, it is time to figure out who you are and what you want to accomplish. With a little flexibility and a few accommodations, there is no reason why plans can't be made for your future for both family and career.

As far as family is concerned, engagements, weddings, and births have all been planned and celebrated by UC and CD patients, and there is no reason why you can't do these things as well, given the right conditions. By the same token, sad happenings such as divorces and deaths have been survived, and you will get through those as well.

Your career may experience a slowdown or a detour due to your disease, depending on the type of job you have and severity of your symptoms. But that doesn't mean you are a failure. It just means that you have had to make accommodations for your illness. Instead, change your direction as well as your definition of success.

When I first started out as a writer, my goal was to make it to *The New York Times* as a staff writer, a lofty goal for a twenty-year-old to have. I finished school, did internships, and got jobs as a staff writer for a few small newspapers until fate played its role and the disease was diagnosed. Even with the diagnosis, I continued to work, finally garnering a job as an assistant in the Detroit bureau of the *Times*. I learned there that many of the writers outside the bureau, while working at the finest publication in the world, led fairly miserable lives. My goal changed. I wanted a life marked by a balance of friends and family, where I had the ability to adjust my schedule for children and illness if need be. I finally went on my own, becoming a freelance writer. By doing so, I redefined what success meant; it was no longer a position but a life truly lived. I also charted a new course on which I have been extremely pleased.

There is similar room in nearly every profession for people to make adjustments of their goals and their definitions of career, life needs, and successes. It takes a bit of creative thinking and maybe a little lean living for a while, but I assure you it can be done.

Make other goals in your life as well. Set goals for travel, sports, volunteerism, and other activities outside of family and work life. On my list when I first wrote this five years ago, for example, was a visit to Paris and a chance to swim with dolphins; as you can see below, I achieved one of those goals on a family trip to the Bahamas. You can do this, too. Write your goals down somewhere and revisit that list occasionally to see how you are doing in accomplishing them. Realize in making this list that your life truly does not have great limitations, and that there is a life waiting for you outside of the disease and living with it daily.

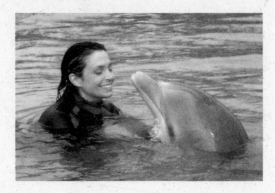

Continue to learn and grow

But just because you are getting busy living doesn't mean you shouldn't also keep tabs on what is happening in the world of research for CD or UC. If you haven't learned to use the Internet yet, now is the time. Check out the research that is going on at the Web sites mentioned in Month 11 and follow the developments. Read other books on the disease. Track down magazine articles about changes in the field of IBD research. Through this education, you are empowered to take on any challenges you may face in the future.

Keep talking to others about the disease. Don't obsess about it, especially if you are enjoying remission. But make a friend on a Web board or at your local CCFA chapter and stay in contact to help each other during remission and flares. Keep talking to your health care team, keeping well appointments and checking in when symptoms arise. Talk to others about the disease to raise awareness.

Your life is moving on, and you are as well. Enjoy it!

IN A SENTENCE:

> *Continue to plan a full and rewarding life, despite the IBD.*

Finding a Cure

ONE OF the goals you can make in defining your future is to participate in the quest for the cure for CD and UC. And the best way to do this is not only by joining but by becoming active in your local chapter of the Crohn's & Colitis Foundation of America.

Since its inception in 1967, the CCFA, formerly known as the National Foundation for Ileitis and Colitis, has established more than forty chapters in the United States that offer support and education services to their members and the communities in which they live. Additionally, the foundation has awarded more than $125 million in research grants to scientists who seek the cause and the cure of CD and UC.

Membership to your local chapter is available for as low as twenty-five dollars per year, with which you annually receive three copies of the national magazine, *Foundation Focus*, copies of your local chapter's newsletter, and reduced price admission to most events.

Raise funds while having fun

Perhaps the greatest amount of local effort is put forth in fund-raising initiatives. Annual Guts and Glory Walks, movie galas, fashion shows, bowl-a-thons, golf benefits, holiday card sales, festive dinners, and other activities help to raise millions of dollars a year. Some of that money stays in the chapter to fund support groups and educational events while the rest of it returns to the national headquarters in New York to be distributed to research grant awardees.

Every chapter has individuals who plan these events and usually there is a need for more to join in this process. Be ready to roll up your sleeves and get to work, but also be sure to have fun as you are sure to meet a lot of people who either have IBD or love someone who does. If you can't plan events, be sure to attend at least one a year to show your support for the chapter. Every little bit helps.

Share your knowledge and support with others

Education and support have been major focuses for the CCFA from the beginning. From seminars to informational meetings to support groups, chapters often offer multiple activities within the year to serve their patient and physician members.

Often, chapters boast education committees whose job it is to brainstorm ideas for new events as well as to coordinate and execute annual gatherings. Ask to join the committee if this interests you, and be sure to contribute your suggestions for events or speakers. The more there are to do the work, the faster the work gets done.

Speak up!

Everyone has the ability to share his or her story in some way or another. Write to your representatives in the congress and senate and petition them for more funding for research of the diseases. Write letters to the editors of your local newspapers during Colon Cancer Awareness Month and pester them about including information about the CCFA and IBD in general.

Someday, there will be a cure for IBD. If we all work toward that goal, that day will be sooner rather than later.

IN A SENTENCE:

> *Get involved in the CCFA's fund-raisers and education and support programs.*

Glossary

ABSCESS: Resulting from inflammation, these cavities tend to collect pus and occur more often in CD patients.

AMYLOIDOSIS: Usually occurring in the kidneys, this extraintestinal manifestation of IBD involves the deposits of certain proteins that eventually interfere with normal renal function.

ANASTOMOSIS: The surgical rejoining of segments of ileum after a resection.

ANKYLOSING SPONDILITIS: An arthritic condition of the spine that is a known extraintestinal manifestation of IBD.

ANOREXIA: A condition that causes less food intake due to an aversion to food or a fear of the pain associated with digestion.

ANEMIA: A low level of red blood cells or hemoglobin, usually related in IBD to intestinal bleeding.

ANUS: A muscular sphincter located below the rectum.

ASCENDING COLON: The right-sided segment of the colon, located between the cecum and the hepatic flexure.

BARIUM ENEMA: A diagnostic test that uses barium as a contrast in the colon.

BILE SALTS: A by-product of the liver that is used in the normal digestive process before being reabsorbed in the ileum; those with ileal disease may suffer from more gallstones and kidney stones as a result of resection or disease not allowing the uptake of the salts.

BIOLOGIC MEDICATION: A relatively new class of drugs, this type of medication targets a specific part of the inflammation process to stop inflammation before it starts.

BIOPSY: A surgical procedure that involves the removal of a small piece of tissue that is later examined by a pathologist for evidence of disease.

BROOKE ILEOSTOMY: A surgical technique used in conjunction with the removal of the colon. The ileum is passed through the stoma opening and folded back on itself before being reattached to the body. An appliance is then used to collect the free-flowing waste.

BYPASS: An infrequently used surgical technique that allows the resected intestine to remain in the body.

C. DIFFICILE: Known more formally as clostridium difficile, the bacteria is a normal inhabitant of the colon that grows out of control when the bacterial balance in the colon is upset, usually due to antibiotic use. It is usually the cause of pseudomembranous colitis.

CACHEXIA: Weight loss that happens during, and is related to, chronic disease activity.

CECUM: The first part of the large intestine, which is located immediately after the ileocecal valve and ends at the ascending colon.

COLECTOMY: The surgical removal of the colon.

COLON: The part of the digestive tract that begins with the cecum and ends with the rectum.

COLONOSCOPY: An diagnostic test in which the physician uses an endoscopic tool to view the colon and take biopsies.

COLORECTAL SURGEON: A physician who specializes in the surgical treatment of diseases of parts of the gastrointestinal tract.

COLOSTOMY: A surgery that calls for the removal of part of the colon and the creation of a stoma in the abdominal wall through which waste exits and is collected in an appliance.

CT SCAN: Otherwise known as computed tomography, this diagnostic test uses computerized imaging to create a picture of a cross section of a patient's body, thus showing abscesses and other irregular developments.

CYCLOSPORINE: An immunosuppressive medication used in the treatment of IBD.

DESCENDING COLON: The left-sided portion of the colon located between the splenic flexure and the sigmoid colon.

DEXA SCAN: More formally known as dual energy X-ray absorptiometry, this diagnostic test is used to determine bone porosity.

DIGESTIVE ENZYMES: A variety of chemicals produced by the body to break down foods into their macronutrients and micronutrients.

DUODENUM: The first segment of the small bowel that is less than a foot in length. It is also connected through the biliary system to the pancreas, the gallbladder, and the liver.

DYSPLASIA: An abnormal development in the mucosa, the presence of which may be a harbinger of colorectal cancer.

EDEMA: The accumulation of fluid in tissues.

ELEMENTAL DIET: A nutrition program used to enhance the nutritional status of individuals who suffer from malabsorption.

ENTEROSTOMAL THERAPIST: An individual who specializes in ostomy care.

ENTOCORT (BUDESONIDE): A rapidly metabolized steroid used in the treatment of disease in the ileum and ascending colon.

EPIDEMIOLOGY: The study of the occurrence and distribution of disease and health related conditions.

EPISCLERITIS: An inflammation of the eye that is an extraintestinal manifestation of IBD.

EPITHELIUM: A layer of cells that lines the intestines.

ERYTHEMA NODOSUM: An extraintestinal manifestation of IBD, this skin condition causes angry red bumps to form on the extremities.

ESOPHAGUS: The portion of the gastrointestinal tract between the pharynx and the stomach.

FISSURE: A somewhat painful crack in the skin that is commonly found in the rectum and anus and can cause bleeding.

FISTULA: A tunnel-like formation that usually begins with an abscess but ends up joining two loops of the intestines or a segment of intestines with an organ or the skin.

FLAGYL: Generic name metronidazole, this antibiotic is commonly used in the treatment of IBD.

FULMINANT COLITIS: A rare and dangerous condition characterized by severe colitis symptoms that can progress to toxic megacolon.

GALLBLADDER: A small, eggplant-shaped sack connected to the biliary system that acts as a reservoir for bile from the liver.

GALLSTONES: Usually made of cholesterol, these crystallized formations are created when there is an imbalance of cholesterol, bile salts, and acids. They are relatively common in CD patients.

GASTROENTEROLOGIST: A physician who specializes in the treatment of the gastrointestinal tract and its associated organs.

GRANULOMA: A nodular lesion present in the intestines of individuals with CD.

HEMORRHOID: A sore bulge in the rectum or anus that is caused by a dilated vein.

HEPATIC FLEXURE: The first bend in the colon, located below the liver and between the ascending colon and the transverse colon.

HEPATIC STEATOSIS: Meaning fatty liver, this condition is a common but relatively harmless extraintestinal manifestation in CD patients.

HYDRONEPHROSIS: Literally water kidney, this extraintestinal manifestation of IBD causes the backup of urine in the kidneys due to the obstruction of the ureters.

HYPERCOAGULATION: An extraintestinal manifestation of IBD, this condition allows for greater coagulation of the blood, leading to an increase in blood clots for some.

ILEOCECAL VALVE: The junction where the ileum narrows to meet the cecum.

ILEUM: The last and longest part of the small intestine and the most common site for CD.

IMMUNOSUPPRESSIVES: A class of drugs used in the treatment of IBD to suppress immune function, thus limiting the disease. Imuran, 6-MP, cyclosporine, and methotrexate fall into this category.

IRITIS: This extraintestinal manifestation of IBD is the inflammation of the iris, the part of the eye that gives it color.

IRRITABLE BOWEL SYNDROME: Known commonly as IBS, this condition is a functional dysmotility of the intestines, causing diarrhea, constipation, or both.

ISCHEMIC COLITIS: A condition in which the blood supply to a part of the colon is cut off partially or entirely. It can cause abdominal pain with the death of the tissue and may lead to gangrene.

J-POUCH: An internal pouch created out of the ileum in UC patients for fecal storage in the ileoanal anastomosis surgery.

JEJUNUM: The second portion of the small intestines, between the duodenum and the ileum, that is about eight feet long in adults.

KIDNEY STONES: A hardened formation of certain salts or calcium in the kidney that can cause great pain as they pass through the ureters and out of the body; CD patients are more prone to these than the general population.

KOCK POUCH: An internal pouch created surgically out of loops of the ileum to hold the intestinal waste in UC patients who have undergone colectomy. It is emptied via a tube that is inserted into the stoma.

LACTOSE INTOLERANCE: A condition caused by the body's inability to process lactose, a milk sugar. It can cause diarrhea, abdominal pain, nausea, and excessive gas.

LUMEN: The hollow space inside the intestines through which the intestinal contents pass. A narrowed lumen may be a sign of inflammation, scar tissue, or cancer.

MESENTERY: A semicircular fold of peritoneum that holds the small intestine in place through a web-like maze of nerve connections and blood vessels.

MUCOSA: The innermost layer of the intestines; includes the epithelium.

MUSCULARIS: The layer of muscle and nerve cells surrounded by the mucosa and the serosa in the intestines.

NASOGASTRIC TUBE: A small flexible tube inserted through the nose, down the esophagus, and into the stomach that is used to either introduce feeding or a contrast solution or suction away excessive swallowed air in the case of an obstruction.

NOD2/CARD15: A gene found on chromosome 16 thought to be related to the formation of IBD in certain individuals.

OSTEOMALACIA: A condition caused by the softening and bending of the bones, usually due to lack of vitamin D absorption.

OSTEOPENIA: Literally bone poverty, this condition is characterized by the reduction in bone density and happens in some people who are on steroids.

OSTEOPOROSIS: Individuals on steroids are at risk for this condition, characterized by a reduction in bone density.

OSTOMY: An operation through which an artificial opening or stoma is created between the intestines and the skin.

PANCREATITIS: Inflammation of the pancreas; can be a side effect of certain medications.

PERFORATION: A puncture or tear in the intestine, potentially allowing the flow of intestinal contents into the peritoneum.

PERINEUM: The natural wall separating the rectum and anus from the female and male genital structures.

PERIPHERAL ARTHRITIS: A common extraintestinal manifestation of IBD, this condition is characterized by swelling and pain in the large joints of the body such as the hips, the shoulders, the ankles, and the knees.

PERISTALSIS: The movement of the intestines to propel contents through.

PERITONEUM: A membranous sac that lines the abdominal cavity, the inflammation of which is called peritonitis.

PERITONITIS: An infection of the peritoneum.

POLYP: A bulge of tissue outward from the normal mucosa. Can be malignant or benign.

POUCHITIS: The inflammation of an internal pouch created in UC surgery.

PREDNISONE: A common steroid used in the treatment of IBD.

PRIMARY SCLEROSING CHOLANGITIS: A complication of IBD, this condition causes the stricturing of the bile ducts and can lead to cirrhosis of the liver or cancer of the bile ducts or liver.

PROCTITIS OR ULCERATIVE PROCTITIS: The inflammation of the mucous membrane of the rectum, usually accompanied by pain and bleeding.

PROLAPSE: The downward or outward movement of the intestines, in connection with a normal or artificial opening. In the case of an ostomy, a portion of the intestines escapes through the stoma. In rectal prolapse, a portion of the rectum escapes through the anus.

PSEUDOMEMBRANOUS COLITIS: A colitis condition associated with antibiotic use and the disruption of the normal colonic flora.

PYODERMA GANGRENOSUM: A painful skin condition that is an extraintestinal manifestation of IBD.

RECTUM: The segment of intestines between the sigmoid and the anus that acts as the last stop for fecal matter prior to bowel evacuation.

RESECTION: A surgical procedure, accompanied by anastomosis, used to remove a segment of intestines.

SEROSA: The outer layer of the intestines.

SHORT BOWEL SYNDROME: Occuring in CD patients who have extensive disease in the small bowel or have had much of it removed due to disease activity, this condition is characterized by poor absorption of nutrients and may be treated with the use of elemental diets or parenteral nutrition.

SIGMOID COLON: An S-shaped loop of colon positioned between the ascending colon and the rectum.

SIGMOIDOSCOPY: A diagnostic test that uses an endoscopic, fiberoptic tool to allow the physician to see inside the rectum and sigmoid colon.

SMALL BOWEL SERIES: A diagnostic series of X-rays used in CD that highlights the small intestines and involves the use of barium as a contrast solution. With the stomach and esophagus highlighted, it is called an upper GI series with a small-bowel follow-through.

SPLENIC FLEXURE: The bend of the colon located below the spleen and between the transverse colon and the descending colon.

STEATORRHEA: Fatty diarrhea that occurs as the result of fat malabsorption. It tends to smell foul and float on the surface of water in the toilet.

STEROIDS: These natural or synthetic hormones help to control water and salt absorption, among other functions; the synthetic variety helps to control inflammation.

STOMA: Greek for mouth, an artificial opening on the surface of the abdomen through which fecal contents escape following ostomy surgery.

STOMACH: A muscular sack that is located between the esophagus and the duodenum. It acts through its own enzymes and acids to break food down. Food is further pulverized by muscular actions before it is passed through to the duodenum.

STRICTURE: A narrowing in the intestines caused by scar tissue.

STRICTUREPLASTY: A surgical technique to widen a strictured segment of the intestines through the opening of the intestines one way, pinching it in the opposite direction, and closing it.

SULFASALAZINE: An anti-inflammatory drug whose use dates back to the battlefields of Europe and which is commonly used in the treatment of IBD.

TOTAL PARENTERAL NUTRITION (TPN): Nutrition that finds its way into the body through means outside the gastrointestinal system, usually through a central or peripheral intravenous line.

TOXIC MEGACOLON: A dangerous and at times fatal intestinal complication of IBD that causes a dilation of the colon and a cessation of normal function; perforation and peritonitis can result.

TUMOR NECROSIS FACTOR: A humoral substance that is a factor in the inflammatory cycle of events.

TRANSVERSE COLON: The part of the colon between the hepatic and splenic flexures, crossing from one side of the lower ribs to the other.

ULTRASOUND: A diagnostic device used in IBD to locate the presence of gallstones or abscesses in patients too ill to undergo other testing.

UVEITIS: This extraintestinal manifestation of the IBD involves an inflammation of the uvea, the vascular layer of the eye.

VILLI: Small, finger- or oak leaf–like projections found in the mucosa, the purpose of which is to absorb intestinal contents.

For Further Reading

Basic IBD medical information

Benkov, K. H., Winter. *Managing Your Child's Crohn's Disease or Ulcerative Colitis*. New York: CCFA/Mastermedia, Ltd., 1996.

Jaff, Jennifer C. *Know Your Rights: A Handbook for Patients with Chronic Illness*. New York: Crohn's & Colitis Foundation of America, 2005.

Saibil, Fred. *Crohn's Disease & Ulcerative Colitis: Everything you need to know*. Buffalo: Firefly, 1996.

Stein, Stanley H., Richard R. Rood for the Crohn's & Colitis Foundation of America. *Inflammatory Bowel Disease: A guide for patients and their families*. 2nd ed. Philadelphia: Lippincott-Raven, 1999.

Thompson, W. Grant. *The Angry Gut: Coping with Colitis & Crohn's Disease*. Cambridge: Perseus Books, 1993.

Zonderman, Jon, Ronald S. Vender. *Understanding Crohn's Disease and Ulcerative Colitis*. Jackson: University of Mississippi Press, 2000.

Psychological support and inspiration

Benirschke, Rolf. *Alive and Kicking*. San Diego: Firefly Press, 1996.

Kron, Audrey. *Ask Audrey: The Author's personal and professional experience in the day-to-day living with inflammatory bowel disease*. 7th ed. Self-published, 1997.

———. *Meeting the Challenge: Living with chronic illness*. 3rd ed. Self-published, 2000.

Kushner, Harold S. *When Bad Things Happen to Good People*. New York: Avon, 1983.

Nielsen, Peter N., Tom Ferguson. *Will of Iron: A champion's journey; a strategy for fitness*. Ann Arbor: Momentum Books, 1993.

Prednisone resource

Zuckerman, Eugenia, Julie R. Ingelfinger. *Coping with Prednisone* (*and other cortisone-related medicines): It may work miracles, but how do you handle the side effects?* New York: St. Martin's Griffin, 1997.

In-depth reading about IBD

Kirsner, Joseph B., Roy G. Shorter, eds. *Inflammatory Bowel Disease*. 4th ed. Baltimore: Williams & Wilkins, 1995.

Prantera C. BI, Korelitz. *Crohn's disease*. New York: Marcel Dekker, 1996.

Diet and nutrition

Janowitz, Henry D. *Good Food for Bad Stomachs: The healthy eating guide for anyone who's ever had an upset stomach*. New York: Oxford University Press, 1997.

Van Vorous, Heather. *Eating for IBS: 175 delicious, nutritious, low-fat, low-residue recipes to stabilize the touchiest tummy*. New York: Marlowe & Co., 2000.

Resources

Crohn's & Colitis Foundation of America
386 Park Avenue South, 17th Floor
New York City, New York 10016
(800) 932-2423
www.ccfa.org

Equal Employment Opportunity Commission
1801 L Street, NW
Washington, DC 20507
(800) 669-4000
www.eeoc.gov

International Association for Medical Assistance to Travellers
1623 Military Rd. #279
Niagara Falls, NY 14304-1745
(716) 754-4883
www.iamat.org

National Center for Complementary and Alternative Medicine Clearinghouse
P.O. Box 7923
Gaithersburg, MD 20898
(888) 644-6226
www.nccam.nih.gov

National Digestive Diseases Information Clearinghouse
2 Information Way
Bethesda, MD 20892-3570
(800) 891-5389
www.digestive.niddk.nih.gov

Revolution Health
www.revolutionhealth.com

UC and Crohn's.org
For teens with IBD
www.ucandcrohns.org

United Ostomy Associations of America, Inc.
P.O. Box 66
Fairview, TN 37062-0066
(800) 826-0826
www.uoaa.org

Acknowledgments

I MUST first begin by thanking the incredibly patient and talented editor, Matthew Lore, without whom the book would not have developed; his assistance and kindness will not be forgotten. Heather Van Vorous, a true friend and the author of *Eating for IBS* and *The First Year®—Irritable Bowel Syndrome*, introduced the two of us, and for that I am indebted to her. Sue McCloskey was also a giant help with her ever-present assistance, gentle prodding, and suggestions. My agent, Janis Donnaud, was tremendously helpful in a variety of ways.

My family was a huge support as well. I thank my husband, Joel, and son, Jonah, for encouraging me and for putting up with my whining and general unpleasantness while I struggled to finish the manuscript on time. You both deserved better but never complained. I love you both more than words can express. Dr. Manny Sklar was a major supporter and helped by reading every chapter and making tremendously helpful suggestions on the copy. I also appreciate his contribution in the foreword. My mother, Kathryn Davidson, has held my hand in the emergency room more times than I can bear to recall. She was a major support to me as I wrote this book as she has always been throughout my writing career and in life in general. She, along with my sister Patrice Rink, sister-in-law Megan Davidson, and occasional interloper Greg Davidson, my brother, gave me respite from writing at our regular Friday lunches as well. My brother, Dr. Paul Davidson, in addition to teaching me how to use a medical library, was able to supply truly odd bits of medical knowledge, and for that I am grateful. My little brother, Eric Davidson, who never thought he could be a cheerleader, was, and I appreciate his encouragement. My mother-in-law, Harriet Sklar, was a peacemaker when Manny and I had our disagreements over text.

I specifically want to single out my gastroenterologist, Dr. Michael Duffy, who has tirelessly worked to improve the quality of my life since that snowy February day we met in 1989. A wonderful doctor, Dr. Duffy was the first to encourage me to expand my medical knowledge by handing me medical papers on a variety of topics, trusting that I was intelligent enough to understand their content. Peter Nielsen has been a great source of inspiration and knowledge as well as a supporter and friend; I remain truly thankful for the day I met him. Audrey Kron helped me to understand that the disease was only a small part of who I am, and for that I am appreciative. I am also incredibly blessed to have had the opportunity to learn from perhaps two of the world's best writing teachers, Anita Lienert and Doron Levin, who gently guided my writing career in the past decade. Their generosity is infinite, much like their talent.

This book might not have been written without the contributions of some fantastic women, including Emily, Lisa Swearingen, Sunni Loring, Cassandra Paschal, Lindsey DeFauw, Lynn O'Brien, Jenny Chicone, Amy Z. Gold, Geraldine Montgomery, Michelle Buchholz, Vickie Manning, Bernice Joyce Gasior, Karen Gauntt, Bonnie Shelleman, and Elizabeth Bolster. Their willingness to share their stories and solutions along with the laughs we shared buoyed my spirit on a number of occasions. Others like Rach Seybold, Jacy Pierce, and Tom also were incredibly generous in sharing their knowledge and experience with ostomies, while Peggy Kagan and Mike Martin shared their children's stories. A special thanks also to Barbara Rosenstein of the Crohn's & Colitis Foundation of America for locating the slides for the manuscript during an especially busy time. She was a lifesaver.

Index

B

bacteria, 5, 22, 94–95
barium, 203
barium enema, 207–8
barium swallow, 202–3
barium X-rays, 24
Bentyl (dicyclomine hydrochloride),
    126–27
bile, 20
biliary system, 81–82
biofeedback, 91
biologic medications, 64, 113–17, 133–34,
    221
biphosphonates, 127–28
black cohosh tea, 144
blood
    disorders of, 85–86
    in stools, 7, 22
    tests, 23, 24–25
bones
    ailments in, 77–80
    Crohn's disease and, 8
    density, 79–80, 140–41, 200–201
    medication for, 127–28
Boniva, 128
bowel cleansing, 178, 204–7
bowel movements, 7, 21, 22
bowel perforation, 66–67
Brooke ileostomy, 183, 185–86, 188–89
budesonide (Entocort), 64, 109, 222–23,
    240
bypass, intestinal, 174

C

caffeine, 159
calcitonin, 128
calcium, 21, 120, 141, 160, 199
Camp Oasis, CCFA, 265
Canasa suppositories, 106
cancer, colon, 22, 25, 194–99
    prevention, 138, 169, 183, 198–99
    screening for, 196–98
    tests for, 207
carbohydrates, 21
carbonated beverages, 160
causes, 3–5
    fatty acids, short chain, 100–101
    food allergy/intolerance, 93–94
    genetic links, 97–98
    infections, 94–96
    MMR vaccine, 96–97
    oral contraceptives, 98–99

    parasites, 99–100
    smoking, cigarettes, 3, 101
cecum, 7, 8, 21
Celebrex, 129
celiac sprue, 22, 25
chamomile tea, 144
childbirth, 225, 226–28
children
    camps for, 265
    daily life, 258–59
    diagnosis of, 266–67
    enemas, administering, 260–61
    growth and development, 268–69
    health care providers, 261
    hospital stays, 263–64
    insurance coverage, 252–53, 264–65
    medication, 115, 259–61, 263,
        267–68
    nasogastric tube, use of, 260–61,
        268–69
    school issues, 262–63
chromosomal links, 4, 95–96, 98
cigarette smoking, 3, 101
cilantro, 144
Cimzia (certolizumab), 115, 221, 240
ciprofloxacin (Cipro), 64, 117, 221–22, 240
clinical trials, 271–75, 277–82
Clostridium difficile, 22, 26, 129
Colazal, 107, 219
cold packs, 78, 89–90
colitis, types of, 8–9, 26, 65–66, 68, 129
colon, 7–9, 20, 21, 138, 172–73
colonics (colon hydrotherapy), 149–50
colonoscopy, 23, 203–7
    test prep, 204–7
colorectal surgeons, 53, 56–57
colostomy, 65, 173, 186
    daily life, 188–89, 190, 192
Compazine, 127
constipation, 7, 22
continent ileostomy, 183–85, 189
coriander seed, 144
corticosteroids, 64, 201, 222
cortisone, 108–11
coworkers, 32–33, 191–92
COX-2 inhibitors, 129
Crohn, Burrill B., 6
Crohn's colitis, 7
Crohn's & Colitis Foundation of America
    (CCFA), 11, 39, 287–88
Crohn's Disease Activity Index (CDAI),
    238–39

Q

Questran (cholestyramine), 126

R

race, 4, 12
rectum, 7, 8, 9, 20, 21
registered dietitians (RD), 57–58
Remicade, 64, 114–15, 220–21, 240
remission, 238–41
research, 118, 270–82
rifaximin (Xifaxan), 117, 222
Rowasa enemas, 106, 219, 240

S

Sandimmune, 112–13
sargamostim (Leukine), 116
scar tissue, 8, 9, 48
serosa, 7, 46, 47
sexuality, 192, 209–14
shellfish, 93–94
shingles, 123
short bowel syndrome, 154
skin, 8, 9, 74–76, 121
slippery elm bark, 144
small bowel series, 202–3
smoking, cigarettes, 3, 101
social stigma, 28, 30, 191–92
Specific Carbohydrate Diet, 94
splenic flexure, 8–9, 21
steatorrhea, 158
stem cells, 116, 118
steroids, 64, 65, 108–11, 141
    bone loss and, 80
    pregnancy and, 222–23
    side effects, 119–23
stoma, 9
stools, tests of, 24
stress, 3, 17
stricture dilation, 170
strictureplasty, 171
strictures, 67–68, 169, 183
    diet for, 164
    surgery for, 170–73, 174
    tests for, 202, 207
sugar, refined, 93–94
sulfasalazine, 105–8, 198, 219–20, 240
supplements
    herbal, 137–38, 143–44
    mineral, 139–41, 199
    omega-3 fatty acids, 141–42
    probiotics/prebiotics, 142–43
    vitamin, 21, 85, 138–39, 160

support, 287–88
    camps for children, 265
    family and friends, 14–15, 17, 28,
        29–31, 178, 258
    groups for, 16, 18, 39–40
    internet message boards, 18, 43–44,
        189
    psychological, 18, 41–43, 192–93
suppositories, 106, 219
surgeons, colorectal, 56–57
surgical treatments, 8, 9, 268
    abscess draining, 169, 170
    bypass, 174
    fistula debridement, 170–71
    need for, 168–69
    resection and anastomosis, 172–73
    stricture dilation, 170
    strictureplasty, 171
    surviving, 178–81
sweeteners, artificial, 161–62
symptoms, 7–8, 22, 47, 48–50
    in children, 266–67
    prior to diagnosis, 2–3
    when to call the doctor, 69–70
synbiotics, 143

T

tacrolimus (Prograf), 64, 113, 224
tai chi, 17, 90, 234–35
tests, 23
    barium swallow (small bowel series),
        202–3
    barium X-rays, 24
    blood, 23, 24–25
    colonoscopy, 23, 203–7
    CT scans, 24, 201–2
    DEXA scan, 200–201
    endoscopy, 23–24, 82
    gastroscopy, 23
    stool, 24
    ultrasound, 24, 201
thalidomide, 224–25
6-thioguanine (6-TG), 112
Th2 response, 99–100
thrush, 123
Tigan (trimethobenzamide), 127
topical medications, 89, 110–11
total parental nutrition (TPN), 155–56,
    174
toxic colitis, 65–66, 68
toxic megacolon, 49, 65–66, 127, 169, 182
transplant, intestinal, 174

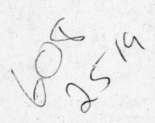